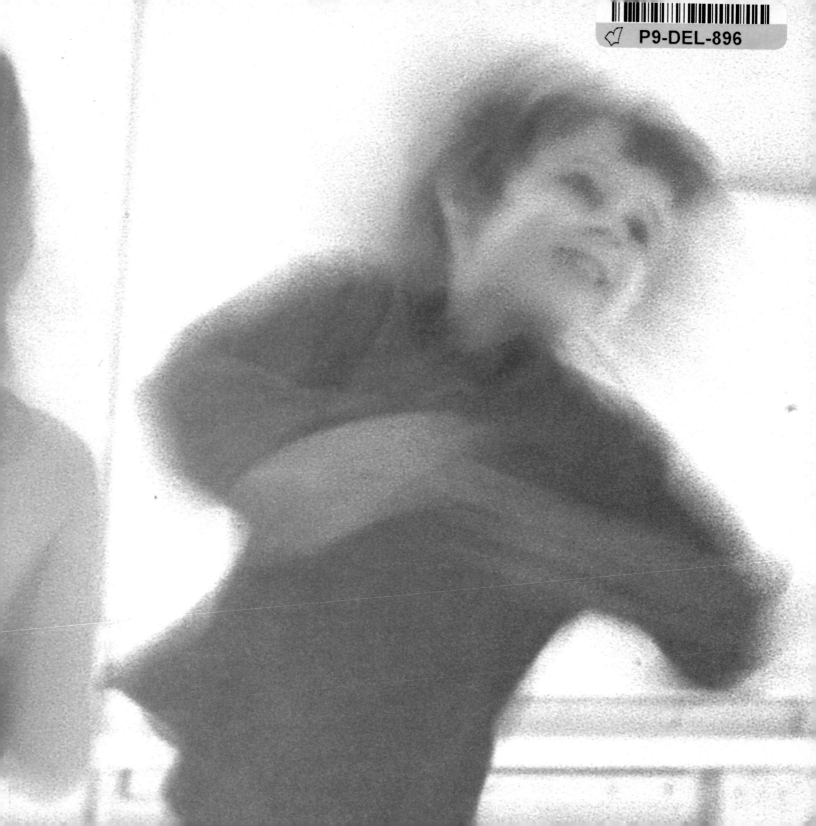

mind mood & FOODS

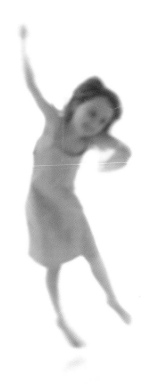

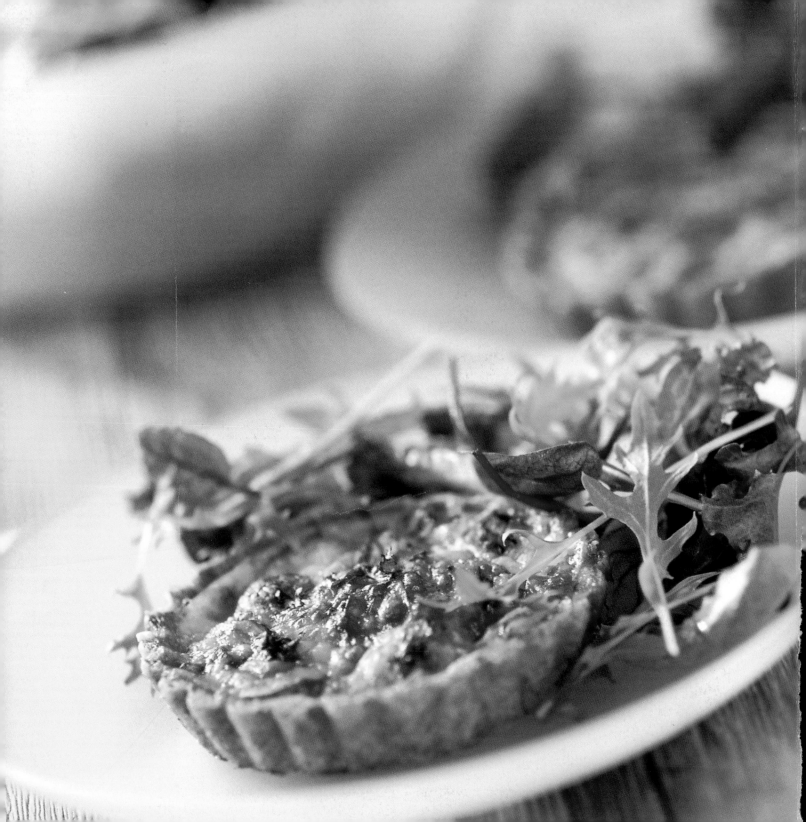

mind mood & FOODS

MORE THAN 100 DELICIOUS RECIPES TO BOOST YOUR BRAIN
POWER, CALM YOUR MIND, AND RAISE YOUR SPIRITS

HAZEL COURTENEY & KATHRYN MARSDEN

RECIPES CREATED BY ANNE SHEASBY

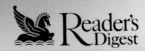

Reader's
Digest

The Reader's Digest Association, Inc.
Pleasantville, New York/Montreal

A READER'S DIGEST BOOK

Copyright © The Ivy Press Limited 1998

All rights reserved.

Unauthorized reproduction, in any manner, is prohibited.

The Library of Congress Cataloguing-In-Publication

data has been applied for.

ISBN 0-7621-0104-0

This book was conceived, designed and produced by
THE IVY PRESS LIMITED

Art Director: *Peter Bridgewater*

Editorial Director: *Sophie Collins*

Managing Editor: *Anne Townley*

Commissioning Editor: *Viv Croot*

Designer: *Clare Barber*

Project Editor: *Caroline Earle*

Editor: *Molly Perham*

Photography: *Marie-Louise Avery*

Printed in China

® Reader's Digest, The Digest and the Pegasus logo are

registered trademarks of the Reader's Digest Association Inc.,

of Pleasantville, New York, USA.

*"Food for thought –
that is what this book
is all about."*

HAZEL COURTENEY

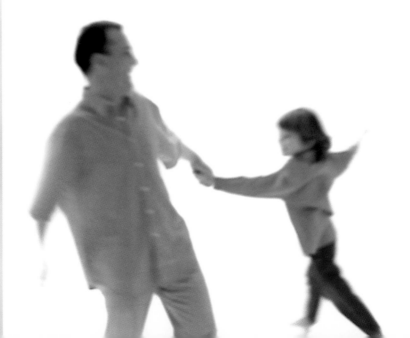

foreword

Until I met my co-author, nutritionist Kathryn Marsden, 20 years ago it never occurred to me that my mood swings, constant tiredness, inability to concentrate, and memory lapses were in any way related to my diet.

Millions of people suffer from similar symptoms, which are often blamed on age, lifestyle, and even the weather. For the most part we accept these symptoms as being part of modern life and put up with them, believing that the way we feel most of the time is normal—but it is not. In Mind & Mood Foods, Kathryn and I encourage you to take control of how you want to feel to suit your unique body and lifestyle. Food for thought—that is what this book is all about. It tells you which foods will help to feed your brain, improve memory and concentration, calm you down, and lift your spirits. It is all a question of balance.

Many people talk about healthy food, but unfortunately in reality continue to eat and drink far too much junk food which depletes vital nutrients from the body and brain. We realize that food alone cannot heal certain mental conditions that require medical attention. But most people, including some doctors, don't realize that the human body is made of food molecules. This includes the brain and nervous system—in other words, we are what we eat.

We do not promise overnight miracles, but if you wish to become healthier and stay that way, you have already taken one step in the right direction by choosing this book. The rest is up to you.

Happy eating!

HAZEL COURTENEY

contents

foreword

5

introduction

8

what are mind and mood foods
and how do they work?

12

notes on ingredients

18

notes on the recipes

19

basic recipes

20

mind foods

22

brain foods

24

memory foods

44

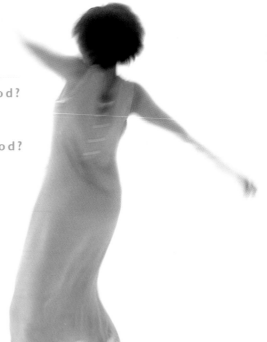

focus foods
64

mental energy foods
84

mood foods
104

relaxing foods
106

sensuous foods
126

feel-good foods
146

reviving foods
166

which mind problem needs which food?
186

which mood problem needs which food?
187

vitamins and minerals chart
188

index and acknowledgments
190–192

introduction

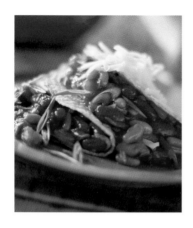

The beans in these tacos provide protein, B vitamins, and zinc—essentials for healthy brain tissue and good memory function.

The secret to maintaining a healthy mind and body is to forget the word "dieting" and think, instead, of introducing some balance and variety into every aspect of life. The maxim "use it or lose it" is true for the whole body, but, as we age, it is especially important for us to keep our mind active. The average human brain contains ten billion nerve cells and weighs about 3 pounds. As the body, brain, and nervous system is made of food molecules, our choice of food has an effect on moods and brain function. In this book Kathryn and I have selected many nutritious foods to help balance your diet toward foods that will improve brain function rather than hinder it. But don't panic—you can still enjoy your favorite treats. I'm sure you have heard the saying "a little of what you fancy does you good"—but note the word little! When you eat chocolate, really enjoy it and don't feel guilty, but remember balance in all things, and keep refined sugary, fatty meals and treats to a minimum.

Today our bodies are bombarded by pollution, food additives, prescription drugs, and chemicals, many of which did not exist 60 years ago, which are now beginning to affect our minds, moods, and overall health. Alcohol and excessive refined sugar, can "fog" the brain, causing a variety of symptoms, depending on the individual. Some people feel tired when they drink alcohol, others become aggressive. We are all unique and this book will help you to find the right foods to suit how you want to feel.

Low blood sugar can cause poor memory and brain function. The secret to controlling blood sugar—and maybe your mood swings—is to eat well-balanced meals and healthier snacks at regular intervals and to be sure you eat breakfast. Above all, reduce the amount of refined sugar you consume in food and drink. Allergy sufferers are painfully aware of how eating the wrong foods can affect their health and we need to remember that the right food is a medicine and a balanced diet is one of the simplest ways to better health.

To survive, the human body and brain need many factors including vitamins, minerals, amino acids, and essential fatty acids, plus air, water, and light. Our bodies cannot manufacture many of these nutrients, so our diet needs to contain sufficient quantities of high quality, unrefined foods in as fresh a state as possible. Because many fruits and vegetables are flown thousands of miles and once harvested can lose up to 50 percent of their vitamin content in just ten days, we recommend you eat locally grown, seasonal, and preferably organic foods whenever possible.

Vitamins, minerals, amino acids, and essential fats from our food work synergistically (together) within the body; therefore you derive greater benefits from eating a variety of whole foods, rather than taking vitamin pills in isolation. Our bodies consist of approximately 63 percent water, 22 percent protein, 13 percent fat, and 2 percent vitamins and minerals, and for optimum health we need to eat a balance of all the main food types—proteins, carbohydrates, and fats.

Protein foods are made from amino acids which improve brain function; they are also essential for muscle tone and growth, healthy skin and nails, for tissue repair, and in the manufacture of hormones. They should make up 15–20 percent of your daily diet. To help wake up your brain, always eat a healthy breakfast, such as eggs or soy milk with cereal or yogurt, which help to reduce food cravings and to improve concentration.

Vegetable-based proteins such as lentils, kidney beans, soybean curd, navy beans, peas, corn, broccoli, scarlet runner beans, and nuts (Brazil nuts, almonds, walnuts, and pecans nuts are proteins) are preferable to animal-based proteins, as they are low in saturated fats and high in fiber. If you are not a vegetarian you can also enjoy fresh chicken and meats (we prefer organic). Fresh fish, especially salmon, tuna, and swordfish, are great proteins rich in brain food such as cholines and essential fats.

Unrefined, fiber-rich carbohydrates such as brown rice, millet, rye, whole-wheat or oat-based cereals, whole-grain breads, pasta, or legumes, and whole foods such as vegetables and fruits contain natural sugars, which help to control mood swings. They also encourage production of the brain chemical serotonin which helps to calm the body and mind. These types of foods should make up 60 to 70 percent of your diet. Sugar is also a carbohydrate and it's worth noting that the foods you tend to eat or crave the most, such as, saturated fats, sugar, and alcohol, are often a contributory factor to your health problems. Foods labeled "low fat" often have a high sugar content, and sugar in excess converts to fat in the body if it is not burned up during exercise. So read labels carefully!

There is also a lot of misinformation regarding fats, and many people believe that low-fat or no-fat diets are healthier. In fact it's the type of fats we eat that are important. Essential fatty acids (EFAs), fats that must come from the diet because the body can't make them, are needed by many body cells to function correctly. Sunflower, sesame, pumpkin, and vegetable oils, oily fish, and avocados are all rich in EFAs.

Many processed foods, such as cakes, pies, sausages, margarine, and burgers contain "hydrogenated" or "trans fats" which should be avoided as much as possible as they cause the arteries to "clog," thus reducing circulation. Avoid fried foods, and use extra virgin oil for stir-fries and unrefined oils for salad dressings. Butter contains vitamin A and although it is a saturated fat, Kathryn and I prefer it to mass-produced hydrogenated margarines. Fat, mainly in the form of essential fats, should make up no more than 30 percent of your daily diet.

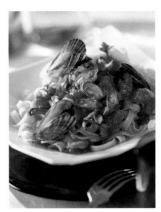

Fish and shellfish contain the amino acid tyrosine, used to make brain-stimulating chemicals that increase mental alertness.

Fruits and vegetables are packed with nutrients and fiber. Try to eat five types every day. Drink plenty of water, avoid excessive use of common table salt (sodium), and take some exercise every day. Learn to breathe more deeply—the mind and body work more efficiently when they have oxygenated blood circulating to the extremities. If we could introduce these ideas into our lives, many conditions such as PMS and mood swings, senile dementia, and even Alzheimer's could be prevented. Nutritional scientists have known for almost 40 years that our state of mind and mental health predominantly depend on the nutrients we absorb from our diet.

Remember, your body is capable of healing itself when given the right tools for the job. Every 72 hours your gut lining is completely replaced, every month your skin is renewed, every year you manufacture a new skeleton and a new liver. Our mind and body strive to maintain a healthy balance, but once a brain cell dies—it's gone forever. Our aim in this book is to help you to look after the few billion you have left and to help to rebalance your mind and moods.

what are mind *and* mood foods *and* how do they work?

PRACTICE MIND CONTROL! *The brain is as dependent on nourishment as any other part of the body. The quality and type of food that we eat can affect the brain's chemical processes, and* consequently influence the way we feel. By carefully selecting what you eat, you will be able to shift your mood, feel more alert, induce calmness, encourage sleep, increase confidence, and reduce stress.

Protein

Proteins are linked to motivation and clear thinking. Protein foods satisfy the appetite for a longer time than carbohydrates and, as a result, keep blood glucose well balanced when eaten in a meal that includes carbohydrates and fats. If you need to be wide awake and in top form, eat a balanced diet that includes protein foods at breakfast and/or lunch. Scrambled eggs, omelet, soy milk, yogurt, cheese, tuna, sardines, all kinds of beans, chicken, and lean meat are all top-class protein providers.

Sometimes, protein foods eaten at night may encourage the brain to be over-active, which may keep you awake. This is because some protein foods contain amino acids, which help to produce brain-stimulating chemicals.

Paradoxically, proteins also contain the essential amino acid tryptophan, which is usually associated with sleep. Milk is often given as a bedtime drink because of its tryptophan content and can, in fact, encourage sound sleep. Tryptophan is needed in the production of the brain chemical serotonin, which has a calming effect. However, although protein-based foods such as poultry, cheese, meat, and fish are rich sources of tryptophan, it doesn't necessarily follow that tryptophan-rich foods will automatically induce calmness and sleep. That's because amino acids tend to "compete" with each other for absorption, often leaving tryptophan last in line. In other words, it may not always be well absorbed. It seems contrary, but a meal containing carbohydrates can be better for increasing serotonin levels in the bloodstream.

Fish and shellfish contain an amino acid called tyrosine, used to make the brain-stimulating chemicals noradrenalin and dopamine, which increase mental energy and alertness. Oily fish contains omega-3 essential fatty acids, which are needed for the production of brain cells. Fish is also a worthwhile source of B-complex vitamins, needed for healthy brain and nerve function. Broiling, quick shallow-frying, or baking are recommended methods for cooking fish.

Yogurt is a great food for waking you up—best for breakfast or as a daytime snack.

Carbohydrates

Complex carbohydrates increase levels of serotonin, the brain chemical known for its calming properties. Feelings of serenity, security, and tranquility are all associated with adequate levels of serotonin. If you are like a coiled spring at the end of the day and need to wind down, it might help to eat brown rice, pasta, noodles, couscous, and potato dishes with your evening meals. Try some of the more interesting carbohydrates such as pasta, corn, rice, and legumes. Complex carbohydrates might help ease anxiety, fretfulness, an over-active mind, irritability, and sleeplessness. A small bowl of granola, muesli or oat-based cereal, or a mashed banana (try it with a teaspoon of cold-pressed honey drizzled over), about an hour before bed might help to encourage a sound sleep.

Serotonin levels drop premenstrually, which may explain why women often feel more stressed, irritable, clumsy, or depressed just before a period, and another reason why they suffer cravings for sweet and starchy foods.

Whole grains such as oats, brown rice, rye, millet, barley, and couscous are excellent suppliers of B-complex vitamins. Oats, usually associated with breakfast foods, are considered comfort foods by some people; another reason why an oat-based cereal could make a soothing snack.

General Guidelines

- If you want to stay awake and alert, eat balanced meals that include proteins early in the day—at breakfast and at lunch.
- If you're feeling down, make sure your diet contains enough protein, but also increase your intake of fresh fruits, vegetables, and legumes.
- If you are anxious, or a worrier, try eating more complex carbohydrates.
- If you want to slow down and sleep, eat carbohydrates.
- If you're under a lot of stress, increase your intake of fresh fruits, vegetables, and culinary herbs.
- Make vegetables and salads a major part of meals, not just a side dish.

Not-so-helpful foods

If you have food allergies or intolerances, or suffer from any gastrointestinal disease, the following foods may be upsetting.

Cow's milk

- Cow's milk is difficult to digest for people suffering from lactose intolerance.
- Yogurt is often tolerated by people with lactose intolerance.
- Remember that many other foods also contain calcium.

Coffee, tea, and cola

- Contain caffeine.

Wheat and yeast

- Tend to be difficult to digest.

Food additives, especially colorings

- While food additives are extensively tested for safety and therefore present few problems, they are generally found in foods of poorer nutritional value.
- Read the labels on prepackaged foods.

Salt and sugar

- Keep salt to a minimum.
- Organic raw cane sugar, molasses, real maple syrup, and cold-pressed honey are flavorful alternatives to white sugar but do not have significantly more nutritional value.

Regular mealtimes

Did you know that the brain has complete priority over the rest of the body when it comes to nourishment? That's why, when we haven't eaten and blood glucose levels have fallen, the first faculties to fail are concentration, information storage, and memory. We're more likely to be irritable, anxious, or suddenly depressed. Eating balanced meals at regular mealtimes helps to keep blood glucose on an even keel, sustaining concentration and coordination. We should include whole grains in well-balanced meals and snacks so that energy-yielding nutrients are gradually released into the system, avoiding fast-release foods such as high-fat and high-sugar fast foods.

Improve digestion and absorption

In order to break down foods that are difficult to digest, more blood has to be diverted to the digestive system. This means that the brain's blood supply is reduced, affecting brain function. One reason why people often doze after a heavy lunch is because the body is working hard on breaking down the meal, and the brain isn't functioning as well as it might.

Tips

- Eat balanced meals.
- Don't prepare huge portions.
- Don't eat on the run.
- Sit down to eat.
- Chew food really thoroughly.
- Leave a few minutes (or longer) between courses.
- Stay seated for 5 minutes or so after the last mouthful.
- Drink a small glass of water or other liquid with each meal.
- Remember to drink water throughout the day.
- If you're rushed and stressed, eat a light snack, such as fresh fruit, salad, or soup, instead of a full meal. Eat a proper meal when you have time to enjoy it. Stress can seriously disturb digestion.

Vitamins and minerals

B-complex vitamins

B-complex vitamins are essential for healthy brain function. A lack of them is known to affect mental processing, perception, judgment, memory, and reasoning. Deficiencies have also been linked to depression, nervousness, anxiety, and low resistance to stress.

B_1

B_1 (thiamin) helps to convert carbohydrates to energy and supports nerve function. A vitamin B_1 deficiency may cause poor concentration, difficulty in recalling information, weakness, low morale, and mental confusion.

B_2

B_2 (riboflavin) is important for energy metabolism.

B_3

B_3 (niacin) is part of an enzyme that helps metabolize energy. Nervous tension, poor concentration, clouded judgment, bad memory, irritability, dizziness, and mental confusion are common features of a lack of B_3. Along with B_6, magnesium, and the amino acid tryptophan, B_3 is needed to produce serotonin.

B_5

B_5 (pantothenic acid) is used for energy metabolism and vital for the support of the adrenal glands. It is also needed for a healthy nervous system. Fatigue and insomnia are classic signs of deficiency.

B_6

B_6 (pyridoxine) is vital for protein metabolism and is known to improve mood. It is also important for immune function and the conversion of the amino acid tryptophan to the neurotransmitter serotonin. Low levels of B_6 can lead to an increase in homocysteine, an amino acid that is associated with heart disease. A B_6 deficiency may cause insomnia, irritability, and fatigue.

B_{12}

B_{12} (cyanocobalamin) helps to ensure a healthy nervous system. A severe deficiency of B_{12} can lead to permanent nerve and muscle damage.

folate

This B vitamin works closely with B_{12}, also with B_6 and vitamin C. A deficiency of folate may cause depression, mental confusion, and fatigue.

choline

Choline is not a true B vitamin, but acts like a B vitamin and plays a role in metabolism. Choline is needed for the production of a neurotransmitter (brain chemical) called acetylcholine and plays a role in memory function. Choline is found in many foods and is especially high in eggs and dairy products.

vitamin C

Vitamin C is well known as a major antioxidant, vital for a healthy immune system and the production of hormones. The adrenal glands store vitamin C and during emotional or physical stress, release the vitamin into the blood. Nearly all fruits and vegetables contain some vitamin C.

boron

Boron is a trace element needed by the body only in the tiniest amounts. It is essential for energy metabolism, a deficiency of boron has been linked with decreased mental alertness.

calcium and magnesium

Although calcium and magnesium are better known for bone and heart health, they are also vital for a healthy nervous system. Deficiencies of calcium or magnesium can have a profound effect on the nervous system.

iron

Researchers are investigating links between iron deficiency and depression, learning, and memory.

selenium

The levels of selenium in food can vary, depending on the selenium content of the soil it was grown in.

zinc

A severe zinc deficiency can impair the central nervous system and brain function.

essential fatty acids

Essential fatty acids are polyunsaturated fats that must be supplied in the diet because the body cannot make them itself. They are needed by every cell in the body and necessary for healthy brain tissue and an efficient nervous system. Vegetable oils, wheat germ, oily fish, meat and all kinds of nuts, and seeds are good sources of EFAs.

Fruit

Fruit is rich in fiber, antioxidants, boron, potassium, selenium, carotenoids, and vitamin C.

apples

- Fiber
- Potassium
- Pectin
- Vitamin C

apricots

- Flavonoids
- Carotenoids
- Vitamin C

bananas

- Vitamin B_6
- Folate
- Magnesium
- Pectin
- Potassium
- Beta carotene
- Vitamin C
- Vitamin B_2

berry fruits

- Antioxidants
- B-complex vitamins
- Iron
- Vitamin C

blackberries

- Fiber
- Magnesium
- Vitamin C

blackcurrants

- Antioxidants
- B-complex vitamins
- Flavonoids
- Vitamin C

blueberries

- Antioxidants
- Vitamin C

cantaloupe melons

- Carotene
- Flavonoids
- Vitamin B_6
- Carotenoids
- Folate
- Vitamin C

carambolas (star fruit)

- Potassium
- Carotenoids
- Vitamin C

cherries

- Carotenoids
- Vitamin C

dried fruit

- B-complex vitamins
- Beta carotene
- Boron
- Fiber
- Iron
- Magnesium
- Potassium

figs

- Calcium
- Fiber
- Iron
- Magnesium
- B-complex vitamins

grapefruit

- Flavonoids
- Vitamin C

grapes

- Flavonoids
- Vitamin C

guavas

- Vitamin C

kiwi fruit

- Calcium
- Fiber
- Magnesium
- Small amounts of iron and B vitamins
- Vitamin C

kumquats

- Vitamin C

lemons

- Flavonoids
- Vitamin C

limes

- Vitamin C

mangoes

- Carotenoids
- Vitamin C

nectarines

- Carotenoids
- Vitamin C

oranges

- Vitamin C
- Folate
- Vitamin B_1

papayas

- Flavonoids
- Carotenoids
- Vitamin C

peaches

- Carotenoids
- Vitamin C

pineapples

- Vitamin B$_1$
- Vitamin C
- Natural digestive enzymes which help to break down other food

raspberries

- Antioxidants
- B-complex vitamins
- Iron
- Fiber
- Vitamin C

strawberries

- Antioxidants
- B-group vitamins
- Carotenoids
- Vitamin C

watermelons

- Carotenoids

Vegetables

Vegetables provide vitamin C, fiber, potassium, and carotenoids. Dark green leafy vegetables can be around six times richer in carotenoids, calcium, vitamin C, and iron than paler varieties.

Yellow, orange, and red vegetables, such as carrots, red and yellow bell peppers, pumpkins, and squashes are abundant in carotenoids (which include beta carotene and lycopene), fiber, phenols (antioxidants), and vitamin C.

The brassicas include Brussels sprouts, all kinds of cabbage, Chinese broccoli, green broccoli/calabrese, cauliflower, and kale. Brassicas supply a few B vitamins, calcium, fiber, folate, iron, magnesium, selenium, silica, sulforaphane, vitamin C, and vitamin E.

Green vegetables are rich in antioxidants, B-complex vitamins, boron, calcium, iron, magnesium, selenium, vitamin C, vitamin E, and zinc. Root vegetables are excellent sources of B-complex vitamins, calcium, and selenium.

alfalfa sprouts

- Vitamin C

artichokes, globe

- Beta carotene
- Folate
- Most minerals
- Naturally diuretic
- Good for the digestion
- Contains cyanarin which is believed to improve liver function

asparagus

- Antioxidants
- Chromium
- Diuretic
- Iron
- Beta carotene
- Vitamin C
- Vitamin E
- Selenium

avocado

- B-complex vitamins
- Magnesium
- Essential fatty acids
- Folate
- Iron
- Vitamin C
- Vitamin E

bamboo shoots

- Trace amounts of calcium, iron, and vitamin C

beans, green

- Vitamin C

bean sprouts

- Iron
- Vitamin B$_1$
- Vitamin C

beets

- Folate
- Potassium
- Vitamin C

bell peppers

- Vitamin C
- Beta carotene

broccoli

- Beta carotene
- Calcium
- Flavonoids
- Folate
- Potassium
- Magnesium
- Selenium
- Antioxidants
- Vitamin C

cabbage

- Selenium
- Vitamin C

carrots

- B-complex vitamins
- Calcium
- Carotenoids
- Fiber
- Beta carotene

cauliflower

- Vitamin C

celery

- Vitamin C

dandelion leaves

- Diuretic

garlic

- Antibacterial and antifungal
- Lowers cholesterol
- Selenium

kelp

- Zinc

mushrooms

- Selenium

onions

- Selenium
- Vitamin C

parsley

- Digestive aid
- Diuretic
- Folate
- Iron
- Potassium
- Beta carotene
- Vitamin C

potatoes

- Vitamin C
- Zinc

pumpkin

- Fiber
- Beta carotene

spinach

- Magnesium
- Beta carotene
- Folate

squashes

- Carotenoids

sweet potatoes

- Vitamin B$_6$
- Potassium
- Beta carotene
- Vitamin C

▪ tomatoes

- Fiber
- Lycopene
- Selenium
- Vitamin C

▪ turnips

- Turnip greens: beta carotene, iron
- Vitamin C

▪ watercress

- Iron
- Vitamin C

▪ yams

- Beta carotene
- Vitamin B_6
- Vitamin C

Fish

Fresh fish is a good source of protein, and nutrients such as B-complex vitamins, calcium, magnesium, selenium, tryptophan, tyrosine and zinc. Oily fish, such as sardines, mackerel, salmon, bluefish, tuna, and trout are rich in Omega-3 fatty acids, vitamin A, and vitamins B_2, B_3, B_5, B_6, B_{12}, folate, biotin, and vitamin E.

▪ salmon

- Calcium
- Omega-3 group of essential fatty acids
- Vitamin A
- Vitamins B_1, B_2, B_3, B_5, B_6, B_{12}, folate, and biotin
- Vitamin D

▪ mackerel

- B-complex vitamins
- Essential fatty acids
- Vitamin A
- Beta carotene
- Vitamin D
- Zinc

▪ seafood

- Chromium
- Magnesium
- Selenium
- Tyrosine
- Zinc

Meat

Choose lean cuts of meat if possible.

▪ beef, lamb, pork

- Iron
- B vitamins
- Protein

▪ chicken liver

- B-complex vitamins
- Chromium
- Iron
- Selenium
- Vitamin A

▪ poultry

- Protein
- B-complex vitamins
- Selenium
- Tryptophan
- Zinc

▪ stock, made with bones

- Calcium

Cereals and grains

Cereals and pasta supply carbohydrates. Carbohydrates are the main source of energy for the body.

▪ barley

- B-complex vitamins
- Magnesium
- Folate

▪ buckwheat flour

- B vitamins
- Zinc

▪ millet

- B-complex vitamins
- Zinc

▪ oats

- Essential fatty acids
- Good soluble fiber
- Iron
- Vitamins B_1, B_2, B_3, B_5, B_6, biotin, folate
- Vitamin E
- Zinc

▪ pasta

- B vitamins
- Iron

▪ rice, brown

- Fiber
- Folate
- Magnesium
- Potassium
- Selenium
- Vitamin B_1
- Vitamin B_3
- Vitamin E
- Zinc

▪ rye

- B-complex vitamins
- Zinc

▪ whole grains

- B-complex vitamins
- Chromium
- Iron
- Magnesium
- Selenium
- Vitamin E

Beans and legumes

Beans and legumes are a good source of protein, B-complex vitamins, iron, and magnesium.

▪ baked beans

- B-complex vitamins
- Calcium
- Iron
- Protein

▪ black beans

- B-complex vitamins
- Calcium
- Iron
- Magnesium

▪ garbanzo beans

- B-complex vitamins
- Calcium
- Iron
- Vitamin A
- Vitamin C
- Zinc

▪ lentils

- B-complex vitamins
- Iron
- Zinc

▪ peas

- B-complex vitamins
- Iron
- Carotene
- Vitamin C
- Zinc

▪ red kidney beans

- B-complex vitamins
- Zinc

▪ soybeans

- B-complex vitamins
- Calcium
- Tofu (bean curd)—an excellent protein source for vegetarians: rich in calcium, magnesium, folate, iron
- Zinc

Dairy products

Eggs, cheese, and yogurt supply the protein needed by the body for growth and repair.

butter

- Vitamin A

buttermilk

- Calcium
- B vitamins

cheese

- Calcium
- Tryptophan
- Vitamin A
- Vitamin B$_2$
- Zinc

eggs

- B-complex vitamins
- Chromium
- Iron
- Selenium
- Vitamin A
- Vitamin D
- Vitamin E
- Zinc

yogurt

- Calcium.
- Yogurt with live and active cultures may be beneficial to digestion and a valuable source of friendly flora
- Magnesium
- Potassium
- Sheep and goat yogurt provides easily digestible protein
- Tryptophan
- Vitamin A
- Vitamins B$_1$ and B$_2$
- Zinc

Nuts

Nuts are a good source of B-complex vitamins, calcium, fiber, iron, magnesium, essential fatty acids, potassium, selenium, and zinc.

almonds

- B-complex vitamins
- Calcium
- Fiber
- Iron
- Magnesium
- Monounsaturated and polyunsaturated fatty acids
- Omega-6 essential fatty acids
- Potassium
- Selenium
- Zinc

brazil nuts

- B-complex vitamins
- Calcium
- Fiber
- Iron
- Magnesium
- Monounsaturated and polyunsaturated fatty acids
- Omega-6 essential fatty acids
- Potassium
- Selenium
- Zinc

cashew nuts

- B-complex vitamins
- Calcium
- Essential fatty acids
- Fiber
- Iron
- Magnesium
- Potassium
- Selenium
- Zinc

hazelnuts

- B-complex vitamins
- Boron
- Fiber
- Iron
- Magnesium
- Monounsaturated and polyunsaturated fatty acids
- Omega-6 essential fatty acids
- Potassium
- Selenium
- Zinc

macadamia nuts

- B-complex vitamins
- Boron
- Calcium
- Fiber
- Iron
- Magnesium
- Monounsaturated and polyunsaturated fatty acids
- Omega-6 essential fatty acids
- Potassium
- Selenium
- Zinc

walnuts

- B-complex vitamins
- Calcium
- Fiber
- Iron
- Magnesium
- Omega-3 essential fatty acids
- Potassium
- Selenium
- Zinc

Seeds

Edible seeds include pumpkin, sesame, sunflower, linseeds, poppy, celery, dill, fennel, and flaxseeds. They contain B-complex vitamins, calcium, essential fatty acids, iron, magnesium, potassium, vitamin E, and zinc.

linseeds

- Iron
- Magnesium
- Omega-3 essential fatty acids
- Potassium
- Zinc

pumpkin seeds

- Iron
- Magnesium
- Omega-3 essential fatty acids
- Omega-6 essential fatty acids
- Potassium
- Zinc

sesame seeds

- Calcium
- Essential fatty acids
- Iron
- Magnesium
- Potassium
- Zinc

sunflower seeds

- Calcium
- Iron
- Magnesium
- Omega-6 essential fatty acids
- Potassium
- Vitamin E
- Zinc

Oils

Oils contain monounsaturated and polyunsaturated fatty acids.

almond oil

- Omega-6 essential fatty acids

cold-pressed oils

- Cold-pressed oils are those such as sunflower, sesame, walnut, extra-virgin olive oil, safflower, soybean, and nutritional-grade linseed oil
- Essential fatty acids
- Vitamin E

fish oils

- Essential fatty acids
- Vitamin A
- Vitamin D

Sugars

Sugars are carbohydrates.

blackstrap molasses

- Iron

honey

- Same nutritional profile as sugar

notes *on* ingredients

Whenever possible, use fresh vegetables, fruit, and juices. Organically grown produce is preferable as it is free from chemical fertilizers. Cooking vegetables by steaming or microwaving is the best way to retain their nutrients.

Organic dairy products—milk, butter, cheese, and yogurt—are available in health food stores and major supermarkets. People who are allergic to or intolerant of cow's milk can use goat's milk, and sheep's or goat's milk yogurt. Although no significant nutritional difference between organic and intensively farmed produce has yet been proved, you may prefer to use free-range lamb, poultry, and eggs.

Oils such as sunflower, sesame, hazelnut, and walnut should be cold-pressed. Most mass-produced cooking oils are processed using heat and solvents. Cold-pressing is a more expensive method, but retains more of the natural goodness of the oil, in particular the essential fatty acids (EFAs) and vitamin E. When a recipe includes olive oil, the best kind to use is extra virgin olive oil. Because it is produced by pressure, rather than by chemical processing, the antioxidants are preserved to give better nutritional value and flavor.

The use of white sugar should be kept to a minimum. Organic cane sugar, molasses, real maple syrup, and cold-pressed honey are alternatives that also should be used in moderation.

Whole grains such as brown rice, oats, rye, millet, barley, and couscous are excellent sources of fiber and vitamins of the B-complex. If bread is to be served with a meal it should be of the organic whole-wheat variety. For people with gluten sensitivity, gluten-free flours and pasta, made from potato, rice, buckwheat, or legumes, are available.

Soy sauce contains some useful minerals, but these include high levels of sodium. Being careful of your salt intake is important if you have high blood pressure. None of the recipes include more than a tablespoon of soy sauce, but some people may prefer to use the reduced-salt version.

notes *on the* recipes

 Spoon measurements used in this book are metric:

1 teaspoon = *5 ml*
1 tablespoon = *15 ml*

The preparation and cooking times are approximate. Ovens and broilers should be preheated to the temperature that is specified in the recipe. The cooking times for all the recipes in this book are based on the oven or broiler being preheated. If using a fan oven, follow the manufacturer's directions for adjusting the time and temperature.

Frozen dishes may be defrosted in the microwave, or left for several hours or overnight in the refrigerator.

Fresh herbs are used in many of the recipes. Fresh herbs give a better flavor, but if dried herbs are used instead of fresh, one tablespoon of fresh herbs is equivalent to one teaspoon of dried herbs. This does not apply to recipes where dried herbs only are listed, such as dried *herbes de provence*, a mixture of rosemary, thyme, sage, parsley and bay leaves.

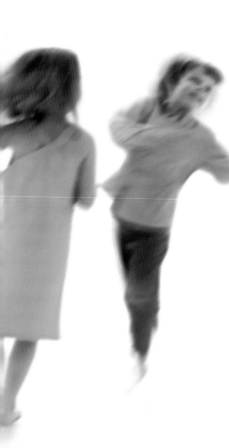

basic recipes

homemade chicken stock

■ ingredients

- free-range chicken bones—fresh or the carcass from cooked meat
- 1 onion or 2 leeks, sliced
- 2 carrots, sliced
- 2 celery stalks, chopped
- 1 bay leaf or 1 fresh bouquet garni

makes approx
3 cups / 1¼ pints (700ml)

■ method

1 Break or chop the chicken carcass into pieces and place in a large saucepan.
2 Add the prepared vegetables and bay leaf or bouquet garni with 3½ pints (1.7 liters) cold water.
3 Bring to a boil; then reduce the heat, partially cover the pan, and simmer gently for about 2 hours. Skim off and discard any scum and fat.
4 Strain the stock through a sieve. When cold, remove and discard all the fat. Cool slightly, then refrigerate for up to 3 days, or freeze for up to 3 months.
5 When required for use, season to taste with sea salt and freshly ground black pepper.

homemade vegetable stock

■ ingredients

- 2 onions, sliced
- 1 large carrot, sliced
- 1 leek, sliced
- 4 celery stalks, chopped
- 1 small turnip or 4 ounces (115g) rutabaga, diced
- 1 parsnip, sliced
- 1 fresh bouquet garni or 1 bay leaf

makes approx
6 cups / 2¼ pints (1.3 liters)

■ method

1 Put the prepared vegetables and bouquet garni or bay leaf in a large saucepan. Then add 3½ pints (1.7 liters) cold water.
2 Bring to a boil; then reduce the heat, partially cover the pan, and simmer gently for 1–1½ hours. Skim off and discard any scum that rises to the surface during cooking.
3 Strain the stock through a sieve.
4 Season to taste with sea salt and freshly ground black pepper.

If not required immediately, this stock can be kept in the refrigerator in a covered container for up to 3 days, or frozen for up to 3 months.

mayonnaise

■ ingredients

- 2 egg yolks
- 2tbsp vinegar or lemon juice
- 2tbsp water
- 1tsp sugar
- 1tsp dry mustard
- ½tsp salt
- dash of pepper
- 1 cup of cooking oil

makes approx
1¼ cups

■ method

1 In a small saucepan, stir together the egg yolks, vinegar, water, sugar, mustard, salt and pepper until thoroughly blended. Cook over very low heat, stirring constantly, until mixture bubbles in 1 or 2 places. Remove from heat. Let stand for 4 minutes.
2 Pour into blender container. Cover and blend at high speed. While blending, very slowly add oil. Blend until thick and smooth. Occasionally, turn off blender and scrape down sides of container with rubber spatula, if necessary. Cover and refrigerate if not using immediately. Use homemade mayonnaise within 5 days.

french dressing

■ ingredients

- 6tbsp olive oil
- 2tbsp white wine or cider vinegar, or lemon juice
- 1–2tsp Dijon mustard
- dash of sugar
- 1 small clove garlic, crushed
- 1–2tbsp chopped fresh mixed herbs
- sea salt
- freshly ground black pepper

makes approx
⅔ cup/¼ pint (150ml)

■ method

1 Put all the ingredients in a small bowl and whisk together until thoroughly mixed. Alternatively, place all the ingredients in a clean, screw-top jar, seal, and shake well until thoroughly mixed.
2 Adjust the seasoning and serve immediately or keep in a screw-top jar in the refrigerator for up to 1 week. Shake thoroughly before serving.

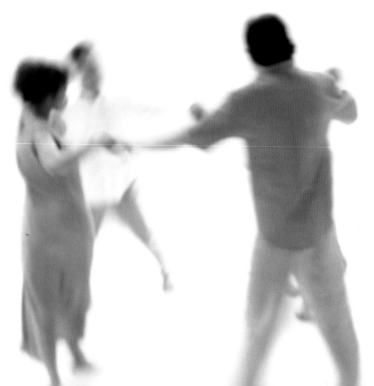

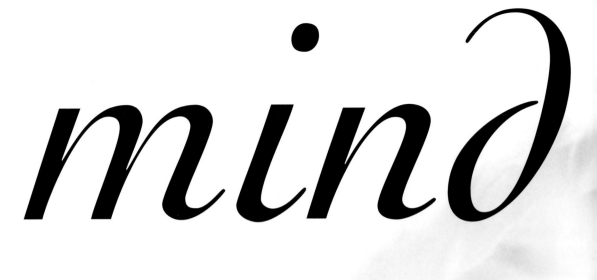

mind

In this Mind section you will find a large variety of foods that will help to feed your brain to encourage a sharper memory, and to improve alertness, clearer thinking, and concentration. For optimum functioning the brain requires plenty of B group vitamins, but vitamin B_3 (niacin), B_5 (pantothenic acid), plus B_6 and B_{12} that are found in liver, eggs, and fish are especially important for clear thinking. Whole grains and cereals such as barley and oatmeal, split peas, brown rice, apricots, mushrooms, and clams are all rich in B vitamins. Essential fatty acids (EFAs) found in oily fish, such as sardines and mackerel; plus nuts, especially walnuts and Brazil nuts, sunflower seeds, pumpkin seeds, and vegetable oils, are vital for the brain development of a growing fetus. Lack of

FOODS

EFAs in some people can affect alertness, memory, and concentration. Lecithin, a substance found in soybeans, other legumes, grains, and egg yolks, is also being studied for its role in brain function. The minerals zinc, boron, calcium, and magnesium plus iron are all important brain nutrients—they are found in seafood, tofu, almonds, sesame seeds, raw wheat germ, dairy products, and blackstrap molasses. Vitamin C, found in citrus fruit, berries, green vegetables, red bell peppers, watercress, and most other fruits and vegetables, aids in the absorption of minerals such as iron, which helps the mind. You will find all these foods and more in our recipes—*bon appetit!*

brain *foods*

THE BRAIN TAKES *priority over the rest of the body when it comes to nourishment. That is why, when you haven't eaten and your blood-glucose level drops, you are more likely to feel irritable, anxious, or suddenly depressed.*

The first faculties to fail are concentration, information storage, memory, and recall. Eating balanced meals and snacks helps to keep blood glucose on an even keel. Choose whole grains and other complex carbohydrates that release their natural sugars slowly into the system.

mixed bean *and* vegetable soup

 This hearty and nutritious soup makes a tasty appetizer or snack served with whole-wheat bread. Beans are a protein food that are also rich in minerals and B vitamins.

ingredients

- 2 leeks, washed and sliced
- 3 celery stalks, finely chopped
- 3½ cups/1 pound (450g) diced, mixed carrots, turnips, and rutabaga
- 1 bulb fennel, diced
- 3½ cups/1½ pints (850ml) vegetable stock (see recipe on page 20)
- sea salt and freshly ground black pepper
- 1 14-ounce (400g) can red kidney beans, rinsed and drained
- 1 14-ounce (400g) can garbanzo beans, rinsed and drained
- fresh cilantro to garnish

serves *six*
preparation time *10 minutes*
cooking time *30 minutes*

method

1 Put the leeks, celery, carrots, turnips, rutabaga, and fennel in a large saucepan with the stock and seasoning and stir.
2 Cover and bring to a boil; then reduce the heat and simmer for 20 minutes, stirring occasionally.
3 Stir in the kidney beans and garbanzo beans. Cover and simmer for 5–10 minutes until the vegetables and beans are cooked and tender, stirring occasionally.
4 Stir in 1–2tbsp chopped cilantro, then ladle into warmed soup bowls to serve.
5 Garnish with fresh cilantro sprigs. Serve with whole-wheat bread or rolls.

variations

• *Use canned green beans or black-eyed peas instead of red kidney beans.*
• *Use chopped fresh mixed herbs or parsley instead of cilantro.*
• *Use 1 large onion instead of leeks.*
• *Use 8 ounces (225g) parsnips instead of fennel.*

freezing instructions

Let cool completely, then transfer to a rigid, freezeproof container. Cover, seal, and label. Freeze for up to 3 months. Defrost for several hours, or overnight in the refrigerator. Reheat gently in a saucepan until piping hot.

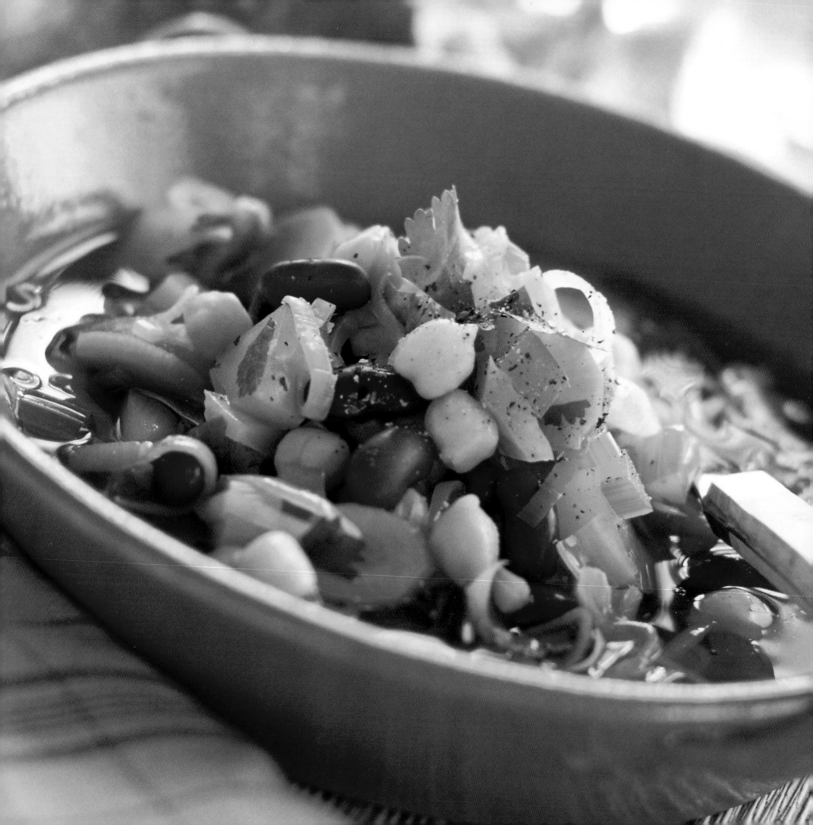

crab *and* corn chowder

This delicious fish chowder makes an ideal appetizer or snack for chilly days. Crab provides zinc, which is needed by the brain for mental alertness, memory, and concentration.

ingredients

- 1 tbsp olive oil
- 1 onion, chopped
- 1 clove garlic, crushed
- 4 celery stalks, chopped
- 1 small green bell pepper, seeded and diced
- 2½ cups/12 ounces (350g) diced potatoes
- 6 ounces (175g) button mushrooms, sliced
- 2 cups/16 fluid ounces (450ml) vegetable stock (see recipe on page 20)
- 1¼ cups/½ pint (300ml) milk
- 1 cup/8 ounces (225g) canned corn kernels
- 1¾ cups/8 ounces (225g) flaked crabmeat
- salt
- freshly ground black pepper
- 2 tbsp chopped fresh parsley
- fresh parsley sprigs, to garnish

serves *six*
preparation time *15 minutes*
cooking time *25–30 minutes*

method

1 Heat the oil in a large saucepan. Add the onion, garlic, celery, and green pepper, and cook for 5 minutes, stirring occasionally.
2 Stir in the potatoes, mushrooms, and stock. Cover and bring to a boil; then reduce the heat and simmer for 15–20 minutes, until the vegetables are just cooked and tender, stirring occasionally.
3 Add the milk, corn, crabmeat and seasoning. Bring back to a boil, then simmer for 5 minutes, still stirring.
4 Add the chopped parsley, then ladle into soup bowls.
5 Garnish with fresh parsley sprigs and serve with whole-wheat bread rolls.

variations

• Use 2½ cups/12 ounces (350g) drained and flaked, canned crabmeat if fresh crabmeat is not available.
• Use canned salmon or tuna, drained and flaked, instead of crab.
• Use frozen petits pois (baby peas) instead of canned corn.

asparagus *with* hazelnuts

Freshly cooked asparagus served with a hazelnut dressing makes a tasty appetizer. Hazelnuts contain boron, a trace element that is essential for normal brain function.

ingredients

- 1 pound (450g) asparagus, trimmed
- ¼–½ cup/1–2 ounces (25–55g) roughly chopped, toasted hazelnuts
- fresh cilantro sprigs, to garnish

for the dressing
- 2 tbsp hazelnut oil
- 1 tbsp olive oil
- 1 tbsp lemon juice
- 1 tbsp honey
- 1 tsp Dijon mustard
- 2 green onions, finely chopped
- 1 clove garlic, crushed
- 1 tbsp chopped fresh cilantro
- sea salt
- freshly ground black pepper

serves *four*
preparation time *10 minutes*
cooking time *8–12 minutes*

method

1 Tie the asparagus in small bundles and cook upright in a deep saucepan of lightly salted, boiling water for 8–12 minutes, until tender. Ensure that the tips are above the water so that they are steamed rather than boiled.
2 To make the dressing, put the oils, lemon juice, honey, mustard, green onions, garlic, chopped cilantro, and seasoning in a bowl and whisk together.
3 Drain the asparagus and untie the bundles. Divide the stalks between four serving plates.
4 Drizzle the dressing over the asparagus and scatter some hazelnuts over each portion. Garnish with fresh cilantro sprigs.
5 Serve immediately with crusty whole-wheat bread.

variations

• Use walnut oil and walnuts instead of hazelnut oil and hazelnuts.
• Use chopped fresh parsley instead of cilantro.

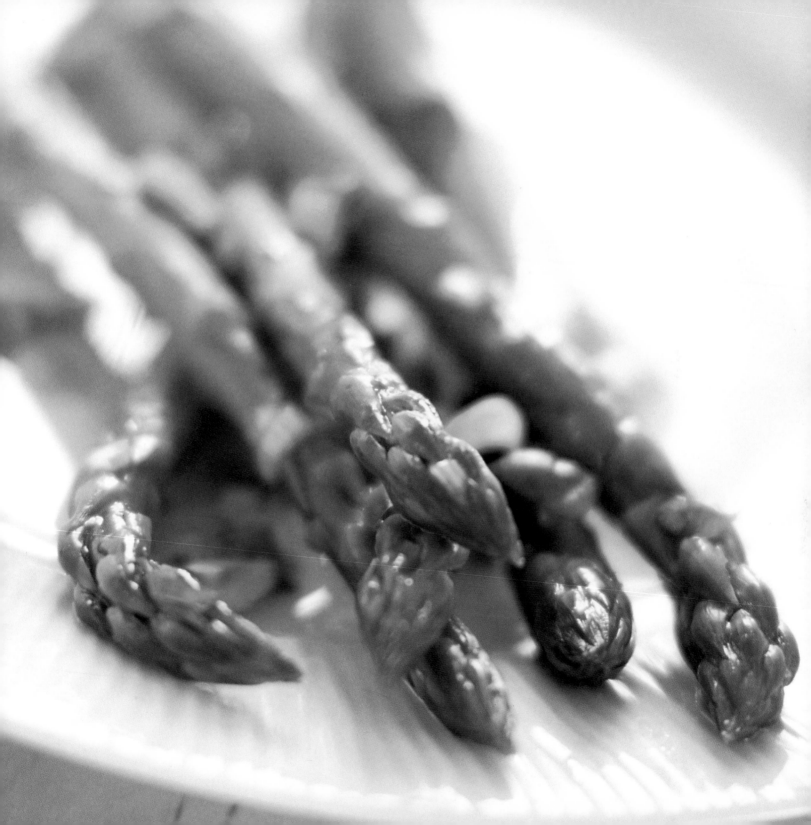

fish *with* broccoli sauce

White fish served with a delicious fresh broccoli sauce makes a nutritious and appetizing meal. Broccoli is a good source of vitamin C, an important nutrient that aids the absorption of iron.

ingredients

- 6 firm white fish steaks, such as haddock or cod, each weighing about 6 ounces (175g)
- sea salt
- freshly ground black pepper
- juice of 2 lemons
- fresh herb sprigs, to garnish

for the sauce

- 8 ounces (225g) broccoli florets
- 1 small onion, chopped
- 1tbsp/½ ounce (15g) butter
- 2tbsp/½ ounce (15g) whole-wheat flour
- ⅔ cup/¼ pint (150ml) milk
- ⅔ cup/¼pint (150ml) vegetable stock, cooled (see recipe on page 20)
- ½ cup/2 ounces (55g) finely grated Cheddar cheese
- sea salt
- freshly ground black pepper

serves *six*
preparation time *10 minutes*
cooking time *20–30 minutes*

method

1 Preheat the oven to 350°F.
2 Place each fish steak on a piece of baking paper. Season, then sprinkle over lemon juice. Fold the paper to make packages.
3 Place on a baking tray and bake in the preheated oven for 20–30 minutes, until the fish is cooked.
4 Cook the broccoli and onion in boiling water for about 7 minutes, until tender. Drain, then blend in a food processor with 3tbsp of the cooking liquid.
5 Put the butter, flour, milk, and stock in a saucepan and heat gently, whisking continuously, until the sauce comes to a boil and thickens. Simmer gently for 3 minutes; then stir in the broccoli purée and reheat gently.
6 Remove from the heat and stir in the cheese; then season to taste and pour over the fish.
7 Garnish with herb sprigs and serve with cooked vegetables.

variations

• *Use fresh spinach instead of broccoli.*

• *Use lime instead of lemon juice.*

cajun-spiced seafood stir-fry

This tasty stir-fry can be served with rice or noodles. Seafood contains an amino acid called tyrosine, which is used to make brain-stimulating chemicals that increase mental energy and alertness.

ingredients

- 4tsp (20ml) cajun seasoning
- 2tbsp (30ml) dry sherry
- 1tbsp (15ml) light soy sauce
- 1tbsp (15ml) tomato paste
- freshly ground black pepper
- 1tbsp (15ml) olive oil
- 2 cloves garlic, crushed
- 2 carrots, cut into matchstick (julienne) strips
- 1 yellow bell pepper, seeded and sliced
- 12 ounces (350g) mixed raw, shelled, prepared seafood such as mussels, shrimp, scallops, and squid
- 2 zucchini, cut into matchstick (julienne) strips
- 1 bunch green onions, chopped

serves *four*
preparation time *15 minutes*
cooking time *8–10 minutes*

method

1 Mix the cajun seasoning, sherry, soy sauce, tomato paste, and black pepper together in a small bowl and set aside.
2 Heat the oil in a nonstick wok or large skillet. Add the garlic, carrots, and pepper, and stir-fry over a high heat for 2 minutes.
3 Add the mixed seafood, zucchini, and green onions and stir-fry for another 4–6 minutes.
4 Add the cajun seasoning mixture and stir-fry until the seafood and vegetables are cooked and tender and everything is piping hot.
5 Serve with brown rice, egg noodles, or rice noodles.

variations

• *Use parsnips instead of carrots.*

• *Use Chinese 5-spice seasoning instead of cajun seasoning.*

• *Use sesame oil instead of olive oil.*

fish *dishes*

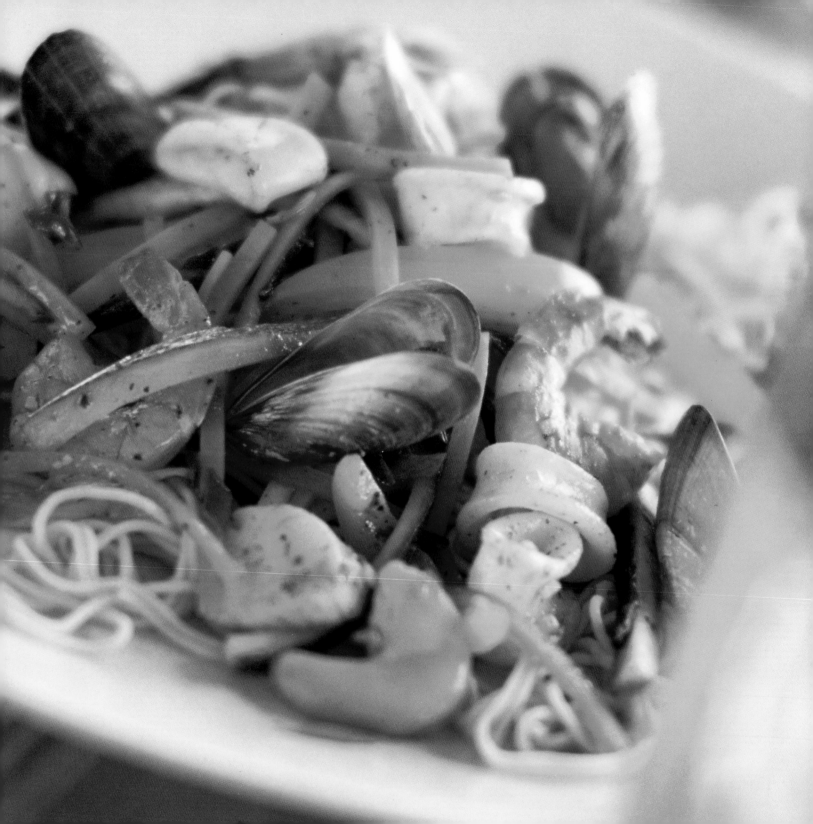

poached salmon *with* celery sauce

 Fresh salmon steaks served with a thick, tasty celery sauce make a tempting dish. Salmon is a good source of omega-3 fatty acids.

ingredients

- 6 salmon steaks, each weighing about 6 ounces (175g)
- vegetable stock (see recipe on page 20), for poaching
- fresh parsley sprigs, to garnish

for the sauce

- 2tbsp/1 ounce (25g) butter
- 3 shallots (French shallots), finely chopped
- 4 celery stalks, finely chopped
- 2tbsp cornstarch
- 1½ cups/12 fluid ounces (350ml) milk
- 2tbsp chopped fresh parsley
- sea salt
- freshly ground black pepper

serves *six*
preparation time *10 minutes*
cooking time *15–20 minutes*

method

1 Place the salmon steaks in a large, deep skillet and pour over enough stock to cover the fish completely. Cover and bring to a boil; then reduce the heat and simmer gently for about 10 minutes, until the salmon is cooked and the flesh flakes when tested with a fork.
2 Meanwhile, melt the butter in a saucepan. Add the shallots and celery, cover, and cook for 15–20 minutes, until the vegetables are tender, stirring occasionally.
3 Blend the cornstarch with a little of the milk, then stir in the remaining milk. Heat gently, stirring continuously, until the sauce comes to a boil and thickens. Simmer gently for 2 minutes, stirring continuously.

4 Stir in the hot cooked vegetables and chopped parsley. Season with salt and pepper.
5 Using a slotted spoon or fish slice, carefully remove the salmon steaks from the stock and place on warmed serving plates. Discard the stock.
6 Spoon some celery sauce over the fish, or alongside, and garnish with fresh parsley sprigs.
7 Serve with cooked fresh vegetables such as new potatoes, carrots, and broccoli.

variations

- *Use tuna steaks instead of salmon.*
- *Use chopped fresh chives or tarragon instead of parsley.*
- *Use 1 onion instead of shallots.*

fish *dishes*

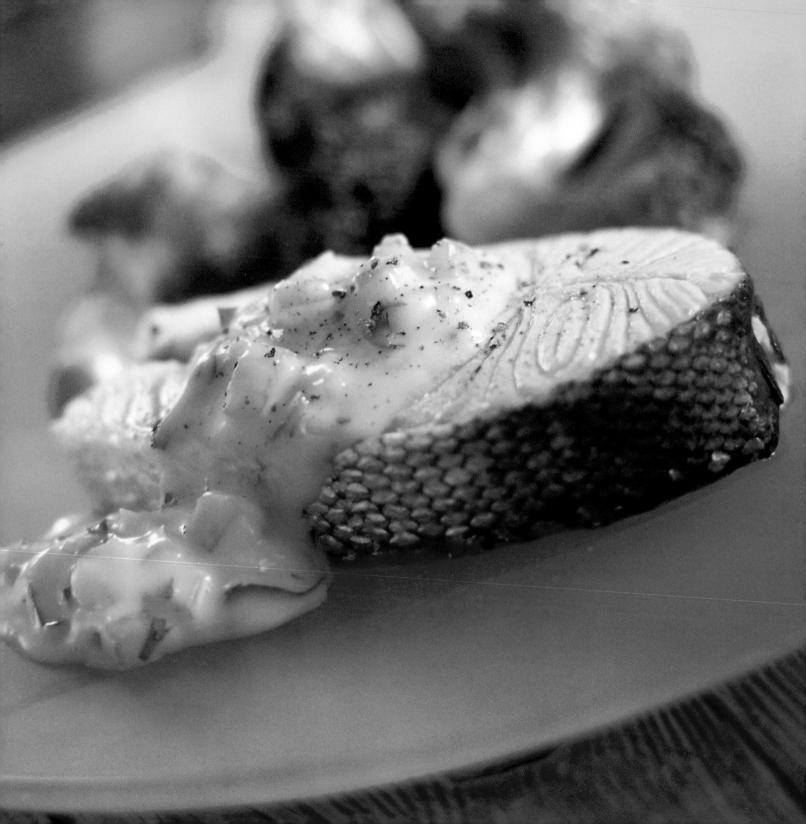

honey *and* mustard chicken drumsticks

 Chicken drumsticks coated with honey and mustard are a popular choice with most families. Protein foods such as chicken contain amino acids that help produce brain-stimulating chemicals.

▌ingredients

- 3tbsp honey
- 2tbsp whole-grain mustard
- 1tbsp olive oil
- 1tbsp fresh lemon juice
- 1 clove garlic, crushed
- sea salt
- freshly ground black pepper
- 8 skinless chicken drumsticks
- fresh herb sprigs, to garnish

serves *four*
(two drumsticks each)
preparation time *10 minutes*
cooking time *20–25 minutes*

▌method

1 Preheat the broiler to high.
2 Put the honey, mustard, olive oil, lemon juice, garlic, and seasoning in a small bowl and whisk thoroughly.
3 Cut three slashes in each chicken drumstick. Place them on a broiler rack and brush each one all over with some of the honey mixture.
4 Broil for 20–25 minutes, until the chicken is cooked through and tender, turning frequently and basting with the honey mixture.
5 Serve hot or cold, garnished with fresh herb sprigs.
6 Serve with oven-baked potatoes and homemade coleslaw.

variations

- *Use lime or orange juice instead of lemon juice.*
- *Use lean lamb cutlets or chops instead of chicken drumsticks.*

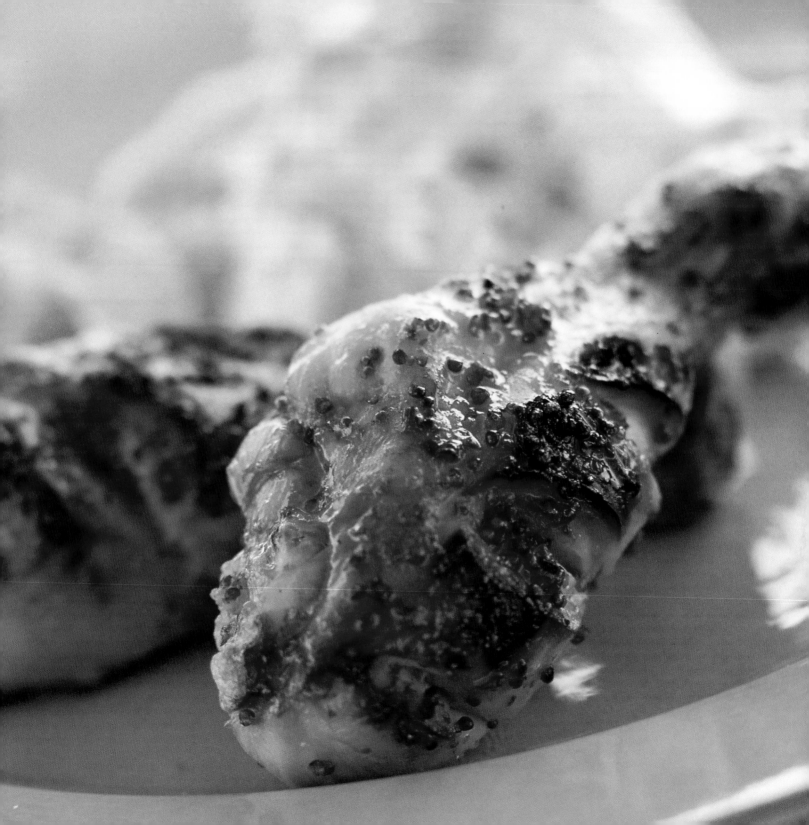

broiled lamb kebabs *with* mint salsa

Kebabs are always popular, especially in the summertime, when they can be cooked over a hot barbecue and enjoyed alfresco. Protein foods such as lamb contain amino acids that help produce brain-stimulating chemicals.

ingredients

- 12 ounces (350g) lean lamb, cut into 1-inch (2.5cm) cubes
- 2tbsp olive oil
- 2tbsp fresh lemon juice
- 3tbsp chopped fresh mint
- sea salt
- freshly ground black pepper
- 1³/₄ cups/1 pound (450g) peeled, seeded, and finely chopped tomatoes
- 2 shallots (French shallots), finely chopped
- 1 clove garlic, crushed
- 1tsp balsamic vinegar
- 1 small red bell pepper, seeded and cut into 8 pieces
- 1 small yellow bell pepper, seeded and cut into 8 pieces
- 16 button mushrooms
- 8 pearl onions, halved
- fresh herb sprigs, to garnish

serves *four*
preparation time *15 minutes, plus 1 hour for marination*
cooking time *10–15 minutes*

method

1 Place the lamb in a shallow, nonmetallic dish. In a small bowl, whisk together 1tbsp olive oil, the lemon juice, 1tbsp mint, and seasoning. Pour over the lamb and mix well. Cover and refrigerate for 1 hour.

2 Put the remaining oil and mint, the tomatoes, shallots, garlic, vinegar, and seasoning in a bowl. Cover and set aside for 1 hour to let the flavors blend.

3 Thread the lamb, peppers, mushrooms, and pearl onions onto skewers. Reserve the marinade.

4 Preheat the broiler to medium. Place the lamb kebabs on a broiler rack in a broiler pan and broil for 10–15 minutes, until the lamb is cooked, turning occasionally. Brush the kebabs with the reserved marinade, to prevent drying out.

5 Serve the cooked kebabs on a bed of brown herbed rice, with the mint salsa alongside.

6 Garnish with fresh herb sprigs and serve with a mixed dark-green leaf side salad.

variations
- *Use skinless chicken or turkey breast instead of lamb.*
- *Use fresh basil instead of mint.*
- *Use shallots instead of pearl onions.*

potato, onion, *and* herb bake

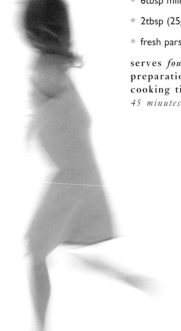 This mouthwatering potato bake makes an ideal light meal. The potato skin adds extra flavor and texture. Potatoes and parsley provide vitamin C, which helps with the absorption of iron, an important brain nutrient.

▌ ingredients

- 1½ pounds (700g) potatoes, scrubbed and thinly sliced
- 2 onions, thinly sliced
- 2tbsp chopped fresh parsley
- 2tbsp chopped fresh chives
- sea salt
- freshly ground black pepper
- 6tbsp milk
- 2tbsp (25g) butter
- fresh parsley sprigs, to garnish

serves *four*
preparation time *20 minutes*
cooking time *about 1 hour 45 minutes*

▌ method

1 Preheat the oven to 350°F.
2 Grease an ovenproof casserole. Add a thin layer of potatoes over the base of the prepared dish. Top with a layer of onions and sprinkle over some parsley and chives, then season with salt and pepper. Continue these layers until all the ingredients are used up, finishing with a layer of potato.
3 Pour the milk over the potatoes and dot the top with butter.
4 Cover with foil and bake for 1 hour, then remove the foil and bake uncovered for another 30–45 minutes, until the vegetables are cooked and tender and the top is lightly browned.

5 Garnish with fresh parsley sprigs and serve with mixed roast vegetables such as bell peppers, zucchini, and eggplants.

variations

• *Use sweet potatoes or a mixture of regular and sweet potatoes.*
• *Use 2 red onions instead of regular onions.*

vegetable *dishes*

warm rice *and* vegetable salad

This delicious salad is packed full of goodness and makes a nutritious light meal. Brown rice, kidney beans, peas, and dried fruit all contain B vitamins, which are essential for healthy brain function.

■ ingredients

- 1¼ cups/8 ounces (225g) long-grain brown rice
- ⅔ cup/4 ounces (115g) frozen peas
- 4tbsp olive oil
- 2 shallots (French shallots), finely chopped
- 1 fresh red chili, seeded and finely chopped
- 6tbsp crushed tomatoes
- 2tbsp red wine vinegar
- 1tsp Dijon mustard
- sea salt
- freshly ground black pepper
- ½ cup/2 ounces (55g) chopped watercress
- 1 red bell pepper, seeded and diced
- 1 bunch green onions, chopped
- ½ cup/3 ounces (85g) golden raisins
- ¾ cup/3 ounces (85g) chopped, ready-to-eat dried apricots
- 1 14-ounce (400g) can red kidney beans, rinsed and drained
- fresh herb sprigs, to garnish

serves *six*
preparation time *15 minutes*
cooking time *35 minutes*

■ method

1 Cook the rice in a large saucepan of lightly salted, boiling water for about 35 minutes, until cooked and tender.

2 Cook the peas in boiling water for about 3 minutes, until cooked and tender. Drain thoroughly and set aside.

3 Heat 1tbsp oil in a saucepan. Add the shallots and chili, and cook for 5 minutes.

4 Put the cooked shallots and chili in a blender or food processor with the remaining oil, the crushed tomatoes, vinegar, mustard, and seasoning and blend until smooth. Set aside.

5 Put the peas, watercress, red pepper, green onions, dried fruit, and kidney beans in a large bowl and stir.

6 Rinse and drain the cooked rice, and stir into the vegetables.

7 Pour over the chili dressing and toss thoroughly.

8 Garnish with fresh herb sprigs and serve with slices of fresh whole-wheat bread.

variations

- *The salad may be served cold.*
- *Use tomato juice instead of crushed tomatoes.*
- *Use arugula instead of watercress.*

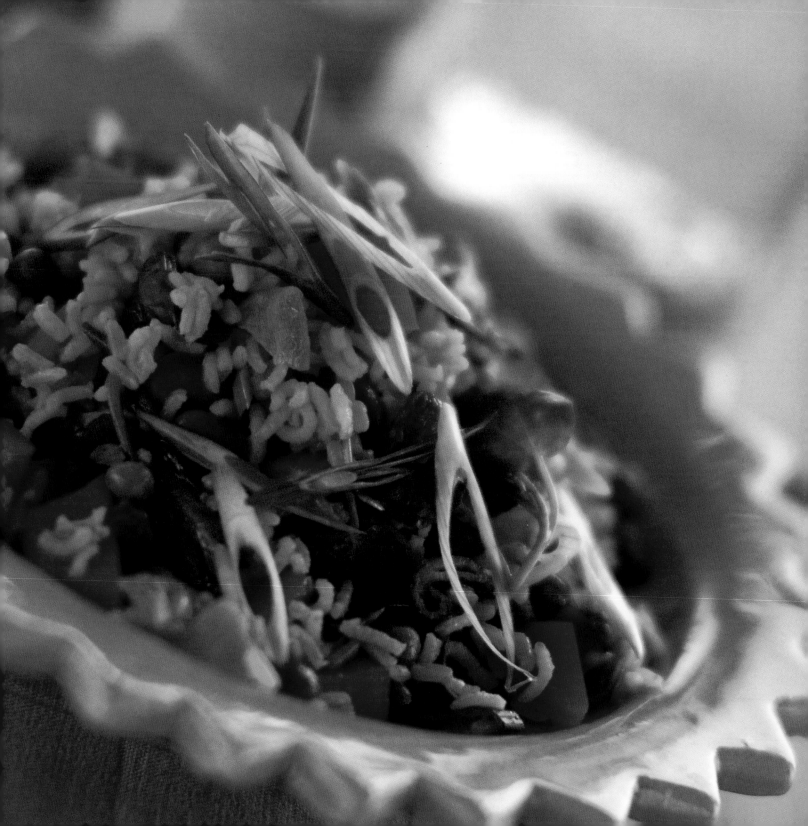

banana *and* pecan muffins

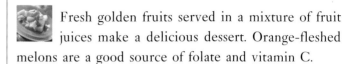

These muffins are quick and easy to make for afternoon tea or breakfast. Nuts provide protein, iron, and other nutrients vital for healthy brain function.

▍ingredients

- 1¼ cups/5 ounces (140g) whole-wheat flour
- ¾ cup/2 ounces (55g) fine oatmeal
- 1 tbsp baking powder
- pinch of salt
- ½ cup/2 ounces (55g) chopped pecan nuts
- ¼ cup/2 ounces (55g) melted butter
- ¼ cup/2 ounces (55g) light brown sugar
- 1 medium egg, beaten
- ¾ cups/7 fluid ounces (200ml) milk
- 1 large banana, peeled and mashed with a little lemon juice

makes *nine*
preparation time *20 minutes*
cooking time *20 minutes*

▍method

1 Preheat the oven to 400°F.
2 Line nine muffin pans with paper cases.
3 Put the flour, oatmeal, baking powder, salt, and pecan nuts in a bowl and stir.
4 Mix the melted butter, sugar, egg, and milk in a separate bowl, then pour over the flour mixture.
5 Gently fold the ingredients together and fold in the banana.
6 Spoon the mixture into the muffin cases, filling each case two-thirds full. Bake for about 20 minutes, or until risen and golden brown.
7 Transfer to a wire rack to cool. Serve the muffins warm or cold, on their own or split and spread with a little butter or honey.

variations

- *Use walnuts instead of pecans*
- *Use ²/₃ cup/4 ounces (115g) dried fruit such as raisins, golden raisins, or chopped ready-to-eat dried apricots or pears instead of the banana.*
- *Use ²/₃ cup/4 ounces (115g) blackberries, blueberries, or chopped strawberries instead of banana.*

salad *of* golden fruits

Fresh golden fruits served in a mixture of fruit juices make a delicious dessert. Orange-fleshed melons are a good source of folate and vitamin C.

▍ingredients

- ¾ cup/7 fluid ounces (200ml) unsweetened apple juice
- ¾ cup/7 fluid ounces (200ml) unsweetened orange juice
- 2 tbsp apricot brandy
- 1 small orange-fleshed melon
- 1 small pineapple
- 1 peach or nectarine
- 6 apricots
- 1 papaya
- fresh mint sprigs or toasted, flaked almonds, to decorate

serves *six*
preparation time *20 minutes, plus 1–2 hours standing time*

▍method

1 Put the apple juice, orange juice, and apricot brandy in a serving bowl and stir.
2 Peel and seed the melon and dice the flesh. Peel and core the pineapple and dice the flesh. Peel and pit the peach or nectarine and chop the flesh. Add the melon, pineapple, and peach or nectarine to the fruit juice.
3 Halve, pit, and slice the apricots. Peel and seed the papaya and slice or chop the flesh. Add to the fruit juices and stir gently.
4 Cover and leave to stand at room temperature for 1–2 hours before serving, to let the flavors blend.
5 Decorate with fresh mint sprigs or toasted, flaked almonds and serve with plain yogurt.

variations

- *Use other mixed fresh fruits.*
- *Use pineapple or white grape juice instead of apple juice.*

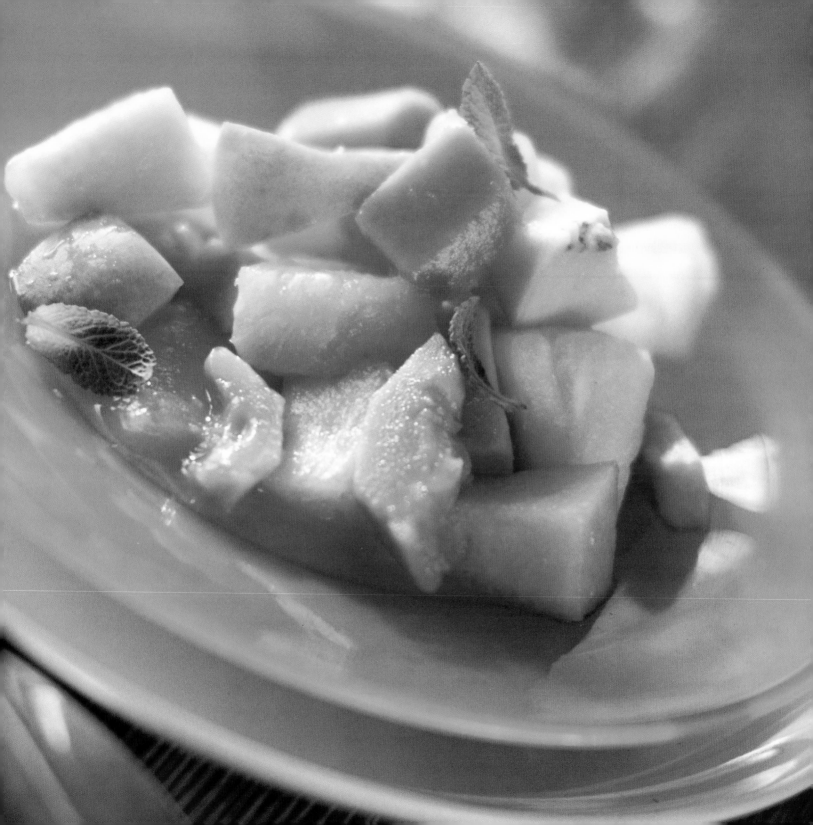

blackberry *and* apple streusel

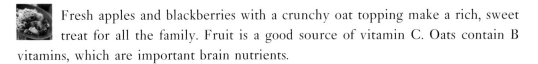 Fresh apples and blackberries with a crunchy oat topping make a rich, sweet treat for all the family. Fruit is a good source of vitamin C. Oats contain B vitamins, which are important brain nutrients.

■ ingredients

- 1 cup/4 ounces (115g) whole-wheat flour
- ½ cup/4 ounces (115g) butter, chopped
- ½ cup/4 ounces (115g) light brown sugar
- ¾ cup/2 ounces (55g) uncooked oatmeal
- 1tsp ground cinnamon
- 2½ cups/12 ounces (350g) ripe blackberries
- 6–8/1 pound (450g) eating apples thinly sliced
- finely grated zest of 1 lemon
- 2tbsp unsweetened red grape juice
- 2tbsp honey

serves *four to six*
preparation time *15 minutes*
cooking time *30 minutes*

■ method

1 Preheat the oven to 375°F.
2 Put the flour, chopped butter, and sugar in a bowl and lightly rub together until the mixture resembles coarse crumbs. Stir in the oats and ground cinnamon.
3 Put the blackberries, apples, and lemon zest in an ovenproof dish and stir.
4 Mix together the grape juice and honey and pour over the fruit.
5 Spoon the oat streusel mixture evenly over the fruit.
6 Bake for about 30 minutes, or until the fruit is cooked and the streusel topping is golden brown and crunchy.
7 Serve hot or cold with home-made custard or yogurt.

variations

• *Use raspberries or blueberries instead of blackberries.*
• *Use ground mixed spices or ginger instead of cinnamon.*
• *Use pears instead of apples.*
• *Use unsweetened apple juice instead of grape juice.*
• *Use chopped nuts, such as almonds or Brazil nuts, instead of some or all of the oats for a nutty streusel topping.*

freezing instructions

Let cool completely, then transfer to a rigid, freezeproof container. Cover, seal, and label. Freeze for up to 3 months. Defrost for several hours, or overnight in the refrigerator. Reheat in a moderate oven until piping hot.

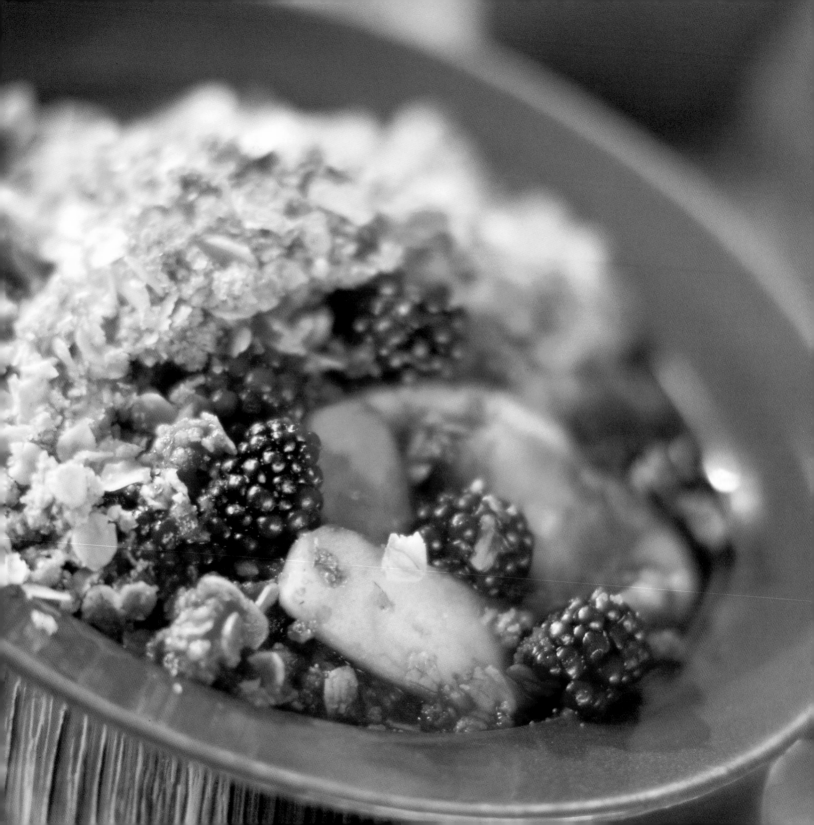

the exam booster

THIS DELICIOUS AND *nutritious menu from the brain foods section is packed with slow-release carbohydrates and protein that will* help *to improve concentration. So instead of burning the midnight oil over a pile of books, sit down to this appetizing meal the night before an exam.*

asparagus *with* hazelnuts

A boron-rich starter—all the better to improve mental alertness.

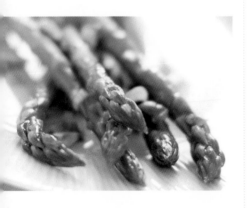

■ ingredients

- I pound (450g) asparagus, trimmed
- ¼–½ cup/1–2 ounces roughly chopped, toasted hazelnuts
- fresh cilantro sprigs, to garnish

for the dressing

- 2tbsp hazelnut oil
- I tbsp olive oil
- I tbsp lemon juice
- I tbsp honey
- I tsp Dijon mustard
- 2 green onions, finely chopped
- I clove garlic, crushed
- I tbsp chopped fresh cilantro
- sea salt
- freshly ground black pepper

serves *four*
preparation time *10 minutes*
cooking time *8–12 minutes*

■ method

I Tie the asparagus in small bundles and cook upright in a deep saucepan of lightly salted, boiling water for 8–12 minutes, until tender. Ensure that the tips are above the water so that they are steamed rather than boiled.
2 To make the dressing, put the oils, lemon juice, honey, mustard, green onions, garlic, chopped cilantro, and seasoning in a bowl and whisk together.
3 Drain the asparagus and untie the bundles. Divide the stalks between four serving plates.
4 Drizzle the dressing over the asparagus and scatter some hazelnuts over each portion. Garnish with fresh cilantro sprigs.
5 Serve immediately with crusty whole-wheat bread.

poached salmon *with* celery sauce

Salmon is a valuable source of omega-3 fatty acids—brain-boosting essentials and important for the healthy growth and repair of cells.

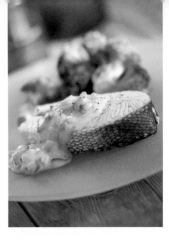

ingredients

- 6 salmon steaks, each weighing about 6 ounces (175g)
- vegetable stock (see recipe on page 20), for poaching
- fresh parsley sprigs, to garnish

for the sauce

- 2tbsp/1 ounce (25g) butter
- 3 shallots (French shallots), finely chopped
- 4 celery stalks, finely chopped
- 2tbsp cornstarch
- 1½ cups/12 fluid ounces (350ml) milk
- 2tbsp chopped fresh parsley
- sea salt
- freshly ground black pepper

serves *six*
preparation time *10 minutes*
cooking time *15–20 minutes*

method

1 Place the salmon steaks in a large, deep skillet and pour over enough stock to cover the fish completely. Cover and bring to a boil; then reduce the heat and simmer gently for about 10 minutes, until the salmon is cooked and the flesh flakes when tested with a fork.
2 Meanwhile, melt the butter in a saucepan. Add the shallots and celery, cover, and cook for 15–20 minutes, until the vegetables are tender, stirring occasionally.
3 Blend the cornstarch with a little of the milk, then stir in the remaining milk. Heat gently, stirring continuously, until the sauce comes to a boil and thickens. Simmer gently for 2 minutes, stirring continuously.
4 Stir in the hot cooked vegetables and chopped parsley. Season with salt and pepper.
5 Using a slotted spoon or fish slice, carefully remove the salmon steaks from the stock and place on warmed serving plates. Discard the stock.
6 Spoon some celery sauce over the fish, or alongside, and garnish with fresh parsley sprigs.
7 Serve with cooked fresh vegetables such as new potatoes, carrots, and broccoli.

blackberry *and* apple streusel

The oats in this dessert provide brain-nourishing B vitamins, and the apples and blackberries are good sources of vitamin C.

ingredients

- 1 cup/4 ounces (115g) whole-wheat flour
- ½ cup/4 ounces (115g) butter, chopped
- ½ cup/4 ounces (115g) light brown sugar
- ¾ cup/2 ounces (55g) uncooked oatmeal
- 1tsp ground cinnamon
- 2½ cups/12 ounces (350g) ripe blackberries
- 6–8/1 pound (450g) eating apples thinly sliced
- finely grated zest of 1 lemon
- 2tbsp unsweetened red grape juice
- 2tbsp honey

serves *four to six*
preparation time *15 minutes*
cooking time *30 minutes*

method

1 Preheat the oven to 375°F.
2 Put the flour, chopped butter, and sugar in a bowl and lightly rub together until the mixture resembles coarse crumbs. Stir in the oats and ground cinnamon.
3 Put the blackberries, apples, and lemon zest in an ovenproof dish and stir.
4 Mix together the grape juice and honey and pour over the fruit.
5 Spoon the oat streusel mixture evenly over the fruit.
6 Bake for about 30 minutes, or until the fruit is cooked and the streusel topping is golden brown and crunchy.
7 Serve hot or cold with home-made custard or yogurt.

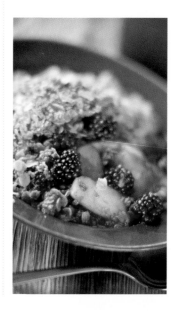

memory *foods*

THE B-COMPLEX VITAMINS *are essential for brain function—a lack of them is known to affect mental processing, perception, judgment, memory, and reasoning. Good sources of B vitamins are broccoli, asparagus, leafy dark-green vegetables such as spinach, bananas, avocados, root vegetables, legumes, nuts,* eggs, brown rice, poultry, meat, dairy products, liver, and fish. Oily fish also contain omega-3 essential fatty acids, which are an important component of brain cell membranes. Zinc is needed by the brain for mental alertness, memory, and concentration. Good sources of zinc are legumes, whole-grain bread and cereals, and fish.*

guacamole *with* vegetable crudités

Guacamole is quick and easy to make for a popular appetizer or snack, served with fresh vegetable crudités. Avocados contain B vitamins and essential fatty acids, which are important for maintaining healthy brain tissue and memory.

ingredients

- 2 ripe avocados
- juice of 1 small lime
- 3 shallots (French shallots), finely chopped
- 2 plum (Roma) tomatoes, peeled, seeded, and finely chopped
- 1 fresh green chili, seeded and finely chopped
- 1 clove garlic, crushed
- 1 tbsp chopped fresh cilantro
- sea salt
- freshly ground black pepper
- fresh cilantro sprigs, to garnish
- prepared vegetable crudités, including carrot, cucumber and bell pepper sticks, baby corn, cauliflower florets, cherry tomatoes, and green onions

serves *four to six*
preparation time *10 minutes*

method

1 Peel and pit the avocados and put the flesh in a bowl. Mash the avocado flesh with the lime juice until smooth.

2 Stir in the shallots, tomatoes, chili, garlic, chopped cilantro, and seasoning.

3 Transfer the mixture to a serving dish. Garnish with fresh cilantro sprigs and serve immediately with a selection of raw vegetable crudités alongside.

variations

- *Use lemon juice instead of lime.*
- *Use regular tomatoes instead of plum tomatoes.*
- *Use chopped fresh flat-leaf parsley instead of cilantro.*

soups *and* appetizers

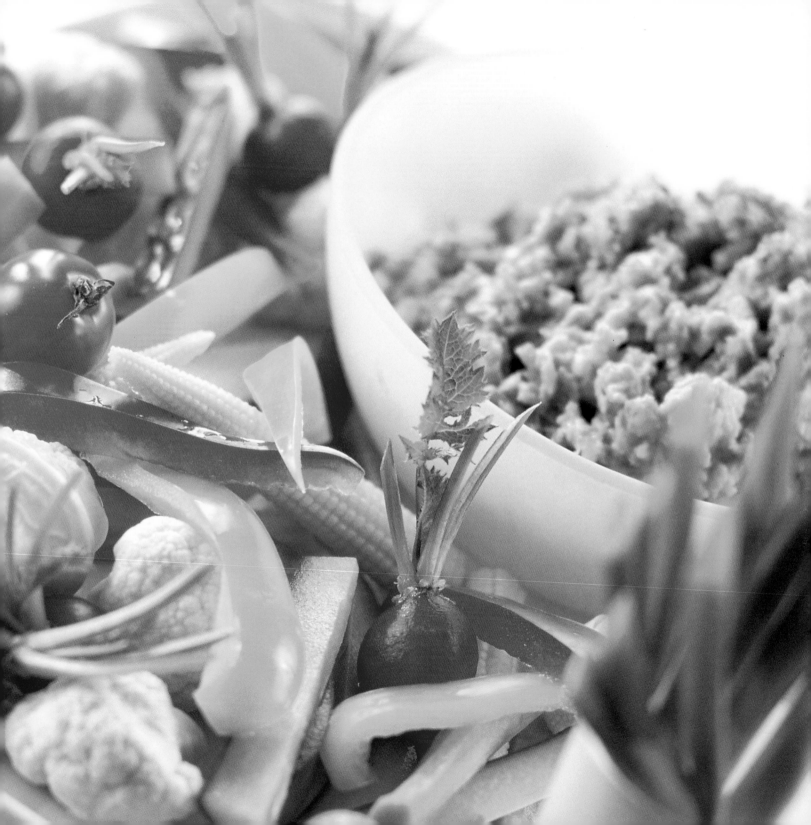

chicken liver *and* brandy paté

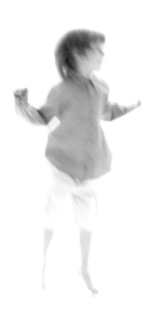 Served with fresh toast or crispbread, this tasty chicken liver pâté makes a tempting appetizer or snack. Chicken livers are a good source of B vitamins, which are essential for a healthy brain and memory.

ingredients

- 1tbsp olive oil
- 1 small onion, chopped
- 1 clove garlic, crushed
- 12 ounces (350g) chicken liver, cut into thin strips
- 3tbsp crème fraîche or light sour cream
- 2tbsp brandy
- 1tbsp tomato paste
- 2tbsp chopped fresh flat-leaf parsley
- sea salt
- freshly ground black pepper
- fresh flat-leaf parsley sprigs, to garnish

serves *six*
preparation time *15 minutes, plus chilling time*
cooking time *10 minutes*

method

1 Heat the oil in a nonstick saucepan. Add the onion and garlic and cook for 5 minutes, stirring occasionally.
2 Add the liver and cook for about 5 minutes, until cooked and tender, stirring frequently.
3 Remove the pan from the heat and cool slightly; then stir in the crème fraîche, brandy, tomato paste, chopped parsley, and seasoning.
4 Put the mixture in a blender or food processor and blend until smooth. Transfer to a serving dish; and let cool; then cover and chill in the refrigerator before serving.
5 Garnish with fresh parsley sprigs and serve with whole-wheat toast or crispbread.

variations

• *Use ruby port instead of brandy.*
• *Use 3 shallots (French shallots) instead of the onion.*

baked eggs *with* mushrooms

Eggs, lightly oven-baked in a nest of vegetables, make a tasty appetizer or snack. Eggs are a source of B vitamins and zinc, which are nutrients needed by the brain for memory and recall.

■ ingredients

- 1 tbsp olive oil
- 1¼ cups/4 ounces (115g) finely chopped mushrooms
- 1 small zucchini, finely chopped
- 1 small yellow bell pepper, seeded and finely chopped
- 1 plum (Roma) tomato, seeded and finely chopped
- 1 clove garlic, crushed
- 1 tbsp chopped fresh chives
- sea salt
- freshly ground black pepper
- 4 medium eggs
- fresh chives, to garnish

serves *four*
preparation time *20 minutes*
cooking time *10–15 minutes*

■ method

1 Preheat the oven to 350°F.
2 Heat the oil in a saucepan and add the mushrooms, zucchini, pepper, tomato, and garlic. Cover and cook for about 10 minutes, until the vegetables are cooked and tender, stirring.
3 Drain off and discard the excess juices, then stir in the chives and season to taste.
4 Spoon some of the vegetable mixture into four ramekins or individual ovenproof glass dishes and make a well in the center of each.
5 Break an egg into the center of each vegetable nest. Cover the top of the dishes with foil and place them alongside each other in a shallow baking pan.
6 Pour in enough hot water to come halfway up the sides of the dishes. Bake in a preheated oven for 10–15 minutes, until the eggs are cooked and set.
7 Garnish with fresh chives and serve immediately with whole-wheat bread rolls.

variations

· *Use fresh wild (field) mushrooms instead of regular mushrooms.*
· *Use 1 red or green bell pepper instead of yellow bell pepper.*
· *Use chopped fresh mixed herbs or parsley instead of chives.*

fish baked *with* lime *and* cilantro

White fish fillets are delicious baked with lime and fresh cilantro. Fish contains B vitamins and an amino acid called tyrosine, both of which are important for the memory and for healthy brain function.

ingredients

- 4 firm white fish fillets, such as haddock or cod, each weighing about 6 ounces (175g)
- juice of 2 limes
- 2tsp finely grated lime rind
- 2–3tbsp chopped fresh cilantro
- sea salt
- freshly ground black pepper
- 1tbsp (15g) butter
- fresh cilantro sprigs, to garnish

serves *four*
preparation time *10 minutes*
cooking time *20–30 minutes*

method

1 Preheat the oven to 350°F.
2 Put the fish fillets in a shallow ovenproof dish. Drizzle the lime juice over the fish and sprinkle the lime rind, chopped cilantro, and seasoning over the top. Dot each fish fillet with a little butter.
3 Cover and bake in the preheated oven for 20–30 minutes, until the fish is cooked and the flesh flakes when tested with a fork.
4 Put the fish fillets on warmed serving plates and garnish with fresh cilantro sprigs.
5 Serve with cooked fresh vegetables such as sugar-snap peas, and rutabaga.

variations

- Use lemons instead of limes.
- Use chopped fresh parsley or mixed herbs instead of cilantro.
- Use fresh salmon or tuna steaks instead of white fish.

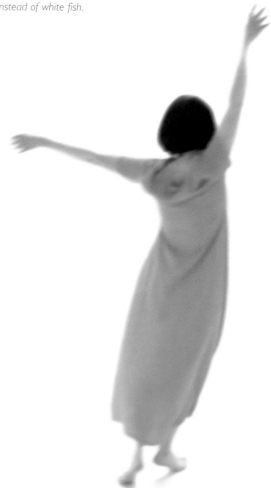

fish

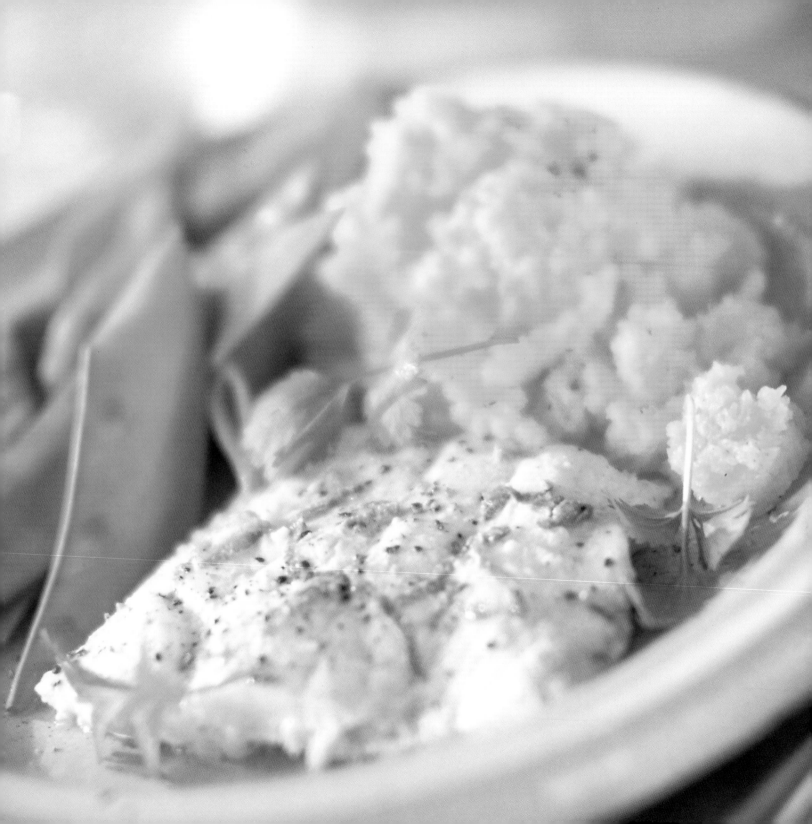

broiled mackerel *with* watercress mayonnaise

Fresh mackerel, broiled and served with watercress mayonnaise, make a delicious lunch or snack. Oily fish are an excellent source of essential fatty acids and zinc, both of which are needed for the production of brain cells.

ingredients

- 8tbsp mayonnaise (see recipe on page 21)
- ¹/₂ cup/2 ounces (55g) finely chopped watercress
- ½tsp freshly grated hot horseradish
- sea salt
- freshly ground black pepper
- 1¹/₂ pounds (700g) small mackerel, gutted and cleaned
- 1tbsp olive oil
- juice of 1 small lemon
- 1–2tbsp chopped fresh mixed herbs
- small fresh watercress sprigs, to garnish

serves *four*
preparation time *15 minutes*
cooking time *8–14 minutes*

method

1 Put the mayonnaise, chopped watercress, and horseradish in a small bowl and mix well. Season to taste with salt and pepper, then cover and refrigerate.
2 Preheat the broiler to high. Cover a broil rack with foil and place the mackerel on the prepared broiler rack.
3 Put the oil, lemon juice, chopped herbs, and seasoning in a bowl and mix thoroughly. Lightly brush the mackerel all over with the oil mixture.
4 Broil the mackerel for about 4–7 minutes on each side, until they are cooked, turning once.
5 Serve the hot mackerel with the watercress mayonnaise spooned alongside. Garnish with fresh watercress sprigs.
6 Serve with whole-wheat bread and a tomato, pepper, and onion salad.

variations

- *Use other small oily fish instead of mackerel.*
- *Use chopped fresh parsley instead of mixed herbs.*
- *Use fresh lime juice instead of lemon juice.*

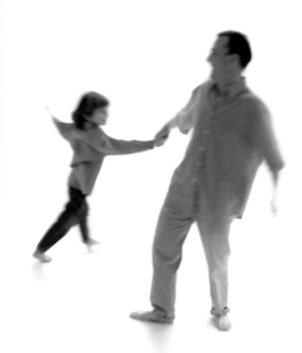

fish *dishes*

stir-fried lamb *with* garlic *and* ginger

This nutritious stir-fry is quick and easy to prepare. The protein contained in lamb encourages the production of brain-stimulating chemicals. Sunflower and pumpkin seeds contain zinc, which can boost mental alertness.

■ ingredients

- 4 ounces (115g) small broccoli florets
- 1 tbsp olive oil
- 12 ounces (350g) lean lamb, cut into thin strips
- 2 cloves garlic, crushed
- 1-inch (4cm) piece fresh ginger root, peeled and finely chopped
- 2 leeks, washed and thinly sliced
- 2 carrots, thinly sliced
- 1 red bell pepper, seeded and sliced
- 3 ounces (85g) sugar-snap peas (mangetout)
- 3 ounces (85g) bean sprouts
- 2tbsp apple juice
- 2tbsp light soy sauce
- freshly ground black pepper
- 1–2tbsp sunflower or pumpkin seeds

serves *four*
preparation time *20 minutes*
cooking time *8–10 minutes*

■ method

1 Blanch the broccoli florets in boiling water for 2 minutes. Drain thoroughly and set aside.

2 Heat the oil in a nonstick wok or large skillet. Add the lamb, garlic, and ginger, and stir-fry over a high heat for about 2 minutes, until the lamb is sealed all over.

3 Add the broccoli, leeks, carrots, and red pepper, and stir-fry for 2–3 minutes. Add the sugar-snap peas (mangetout) and bean sprouts, and stir-fry for another 2–3 minutes.

4 Add the apple juice, soy sauce, and black pepper, and stir-fry until the mixture is piping hot and the lamb and vegetables are cooked and tender.

5 Scatter over the sunflower or pumpkin seeds, and serve with brown rice or pasta.

variations

• *The juices of the stir-fry can be thickened before serving. Blend 1 tsp cornstarch with 1 tbsp water, add to the juices in the pan, and stir-fry until cooked and thickened.*

• *Use cauliflower instead of broccoli.*

• *Use skinless chicken or turkey breast instead of lamb.*

chicken *and* garbanzo bean casserole

This one-pot dish of chicken, garbanzo beans, and vegetables makes a nutritious and filling family meal. Garbanzo beans are a good source of zinc, a nutrient needed by the brain for memory and recall.

ingredients

- 1 tbsp olive oil
- 1 pound (450g) skinless, boneless chicken breast, cut into 1-inch (2.5cm) cubes
- 8 ounces (225g) shallots (French shallots), sliced
- 2 leeks, washed and sliced
- 1 green bell pepper, seeded and diced
- 8 ounces (225g) mixed cremini and button mushrooms, sliced
- 1 cup/6 ounces (175g) frozen peas
- 2 14-ounce (400g) cans garbanzo beans, rinsed and drained
- 1 14-ounce (400g) can chopped tomatoes
- 1 tbsp sun-dried tomato paste
- ²/₃ cup/¼ pint (150ml) chicken stock (see recipe on page 20)
- 1¼ cups/½ pint (300ml) dry white wine
- 1 bouquet garni
- sea salt
- freshly ground black pepper
- 1 tbsp cornstarch (optional)
- fresh herb sprigs, to garnish

serves *six*
preparation time *25 minutes*
cooking time *1 hour*

method

1 Preheat the oven to 350°F.
2 Heat the oil in a large flameproof, ovenproof casserole. Add the chicken pieces and cook gently until lightly browned all over, stirring occasionally.
3 Stir in the shallots, leeks, green pepper, mushrooms, peas, and garbanzo beans.
4 Add the tomatoes, tomato paste, stock, wine, bouquet garni, and seasoning, and stir.
5 Bring to a boil, stirring occasionally, then cover and bake for about 1 hour, until the chicken and vegetables are cooked and tender, stirring once or twice. Remove from the oven and discard the bouquet garni.
6 Blend the cornstarch, if using, with 3tbsp water and stir into the casserole. Heat gently, stirring continuously, until the mixture comes to a boil and thickens slightly. Simmer gently for 2 minutes, stirring occasionally.
7 Spoon onto warmed serving plates. Garnish with herb sprigs and serve with whole-wheat bread.

variations
• *Use skinless, boneless turkey breast instead of chicken.*
• *Use canned red kidney beans or green beans instead of garbanzo beans.*
• *Use red wine instead of white wine.*
• *Use 1 onion instead of shallots.*

freezing instructions
Let cool completely, then transfer to a rigid, freezeproof container. Cover, seal, and label. Freeze for up to 3 months. Defrost for several hours, or overnight in the refrigerator. Reheat gently in a saucepan or moderate oven until piping hot.

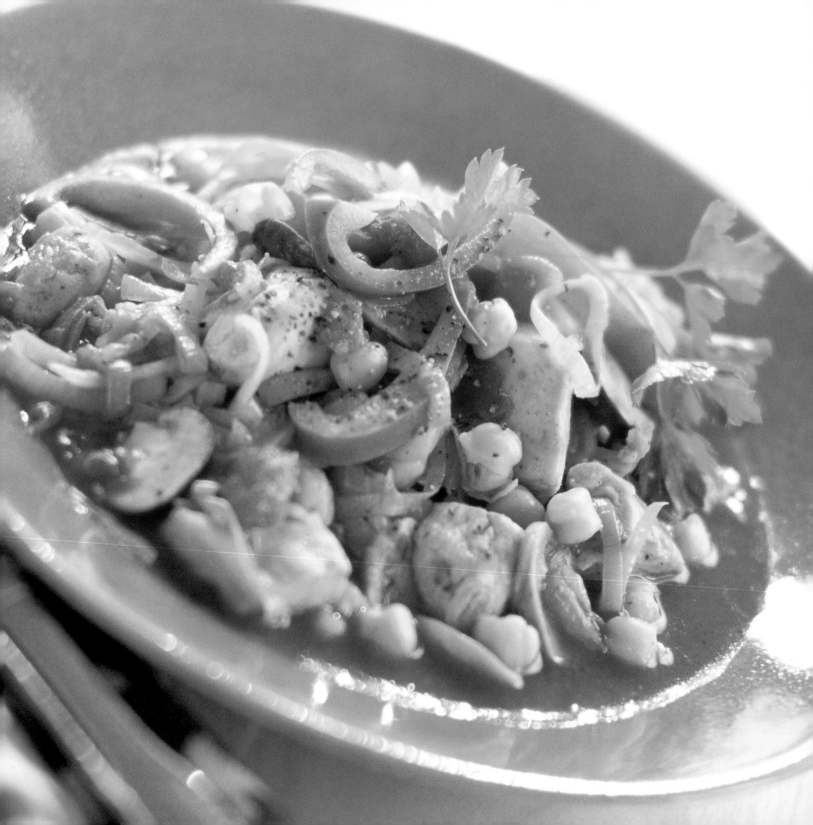

onion tartlets

These tartlets can be served warm or cold with baked potatoes and a side salad. Cold-pressed oil such as extra virgin olive oil contains essential fatty acids, which are important for healthy brain tissue and memory function.

ingredients

- 1 tbsp olive oil
- 1 large onion, thinly sliced
- $\frac{1}{2}$ cup/2 ounces (55g) grated Cheddar cheese
- 2 medium eggs
- scant $\frac{1}{2}$ cup/3$\frac{1}{2}$ fluid ounces (100ml) milk
- 1 tbsp chopped fresh mixed herbs
- sea salt
- freshly ground black pepper
- fresh herb sprigs, to garnish

for the pastry

- 1$\frac{1}{2}$ cups/6 ounces (175g) whole-wheat flour
- dash of salt
- $\frac{1}{3}$ cup/3 ounces (85g) butter, chopped

makes *6*
preparation time *35 minutes, plus 30 minutes chilling time*
cooking time *20–30 minutes*

method

1 Preheat the oven to 400°F.
2 To make the pastry, put the flour and a dash of salt in a bowl, then lightly rub in the chopped butter until the mixture resembles bread crumbs. Add enough cold water to make a soft dough.
3 Roll the dough out on a lightly floured surface and use to line six individual 4-inch (10cm) fluted tart tins. Refrigerate for 30 minutes.
4 Heat the oil in a skillet. Add the onion and cook for about 10 minutes, until softened, stirring occasionally. Remove from the heat and set aside.
5 Line the pastry cases with parchment paper and fill with baking beans. Place on two baking trays and bake blind in the preheated oven for about 10 minutes, until set. Remove from the oven and lift out the paper and beans. Reduce the oven temperature to 350°F.

6 Spoon some cooked onion over the base of each pastry case and sprinkle the cheese over the top. Beat the eggs, milk, chopped herbs, and seasoning together, and pour into the flan cases over the onions and cheese.
7 Bake in the preheated oven for 20–30 minutes, until golden brown.
8 Garnish with the herb sprigs and serve warm or cold with oven-baked potatoes and a mixed salad.

variations

- *Use chopped fresh chives instead of mixed herbs.*
- *Use fresh Parmesan cheese instead of Cheddar cheese.*

freezing instructions

Let cool completely, then wrap in foil. or seal in a freezer bag and label. Freeze for up to 3 months. Defrost for several hours, or overnight in the refrigerator. Serve cold or reheat in a moderate oven.

vegetable *dishes*

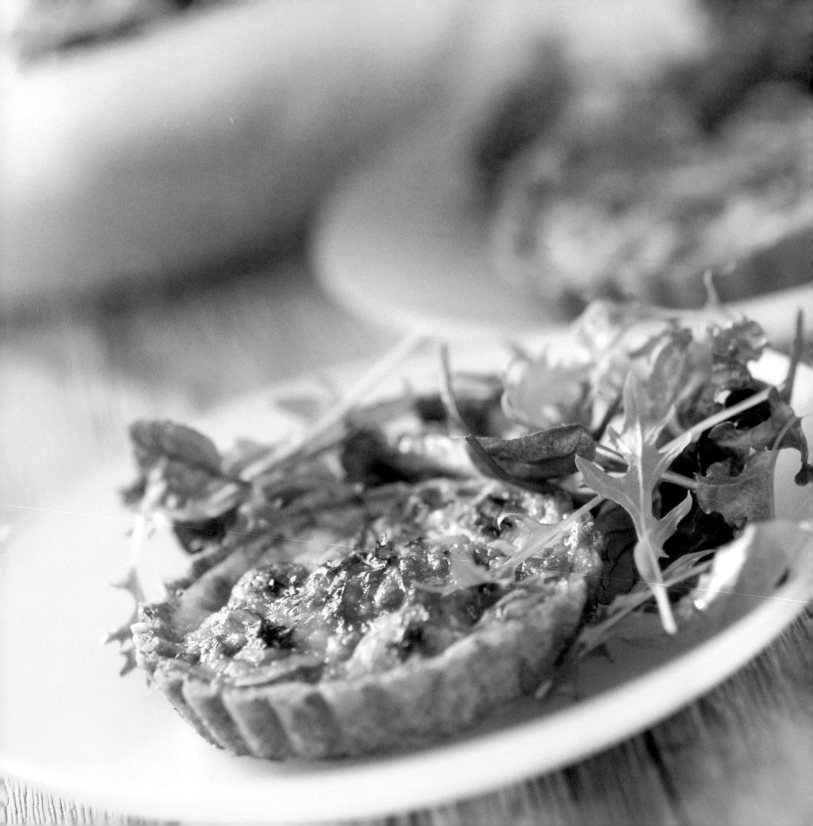

lentil moussaka

This appetizing meat-free moussaka is good served with oven-baked potatoes and cooked vegetables. Lentils provide B vitamins and zinc.

ingredients

- I pound (450g) eggplants, sliced
- sea salt and ground black pepper
- 4tbsp olive oil
- I onion, sliced
- I red bell pepper, seeded and diced
- 2 leeks, washed and sliced
- I clove garlic, crushed
- 2¹/₂ cups/1 pound (450g) cooked green or brown lentils
- I 14-ounce (400g) can chopped tomatoes
- 6tbsp red wine
- I tbsp sun-dried tomato paste
- 2tsp dried *herbes de provence*
- 1¹/₂ cups/12 ounces (350g) plain yogurt
- 2 medium eggs
- ¹/₄–¹/₂ cup/1–2 ounces (25–55g) finely grated, fresh Parmesan or Cheddar cheese (optional)
- fresh herb sprigs, to garnish

serves *four to six*
preparation time *35 minutes, plus 30 minutes' standing time for the eggplants*
cooking time *45 minutes*

method

1 Preheat the oven to 350°F.
2 Put the eggplant in a colander, sprinkle with salt, and leave for 30 minutes. Rinse and pat dry.
3 Heat 1tbsp oil in a saucepan. Add the onion, red pepper, leeks, and garlic. Cook for 5 minutes, stirring occasionally.
4 Add the lentils, tomatoes, red wine, tomato paste, dried herbs, and seasoning. Cover and bring to a boil; then reduce the heat and simmer for 10 minutes.
5 Heat the remaining oil and fry the eggplant slices until browned.
6 Put layers of eggplant and lentils in an ovenproof dish. Beat the yogurt, eggs, and seasoning, and pour over. Sprinkle with cheese. Bake in the preheated oven for 45 minutes.
7 Garnish with the herb sprigs and serve with baked potatoes and broccoli.

variations

• *Use apple juice instead of red wine.*
• *Use sliced zucchini instead of eggplant.*

sweet *and* sour bean tacos

These generously filled tacos are sure to be a popular choice with family and friends. Beans provide protein, B vitamins, and zinc.

ingredients

- I tbsp cornstarch
- 8tbsp unsweetened pineapple juice
- 2tbsp light soy sauce
- 2tbsp light brown sugar
- 2tbsp tomato paste
- 2tbsp dry sherry
- 2tbsp cider vinegar
- I 14-ounce (400g) can red kidney beans, rinsed and drained
- I 14-ounce (400g) can black-eyed peas, rinsed and drained
- 3 plum (Roma) tomatoes, peeled, seeded, and chopped
- I bunch green onions, chopped
- I–2tbsp chopped fresh cilantro (optional)
- sea salt
- freshly ground black pepper
- 8 taco shells
- grated Cheddar cheese, to serve

serves *four*
(two tacos each)
preparation time *10 minutes*
cooking time *15–20 minutes*

method

1 Preheat the oven to 350°F.
2 Blend the cornstarch with the pineapple juice in a saucepan; then add the soy sauce, sugar, tomato paste, sherry, and vinegar, and stir. Heat gently until the sauce comes to a boil and thickens. Add the beans, peas, tomatoes, and green onions. Return to a boil, reduce the heat, and simmer for 10 minutes, stirring occasionally.
3 Stir in the chopped cilantro, if using, and season to taste.
4 Put the tacos on a baking sheet and heat in the preheated oven for 2–3 minutes, until warm.
6 Fill each taco with bean mixture and top with grated cheese. Serve with a mixed dark-green leaf salad.

variations

• *Serve with baked potatoes, brown rice, or pasta instead of tacos.*
• *Use chopped fresh mixed herbs or parsley instead of cilantro.*

vegetable *dishes*

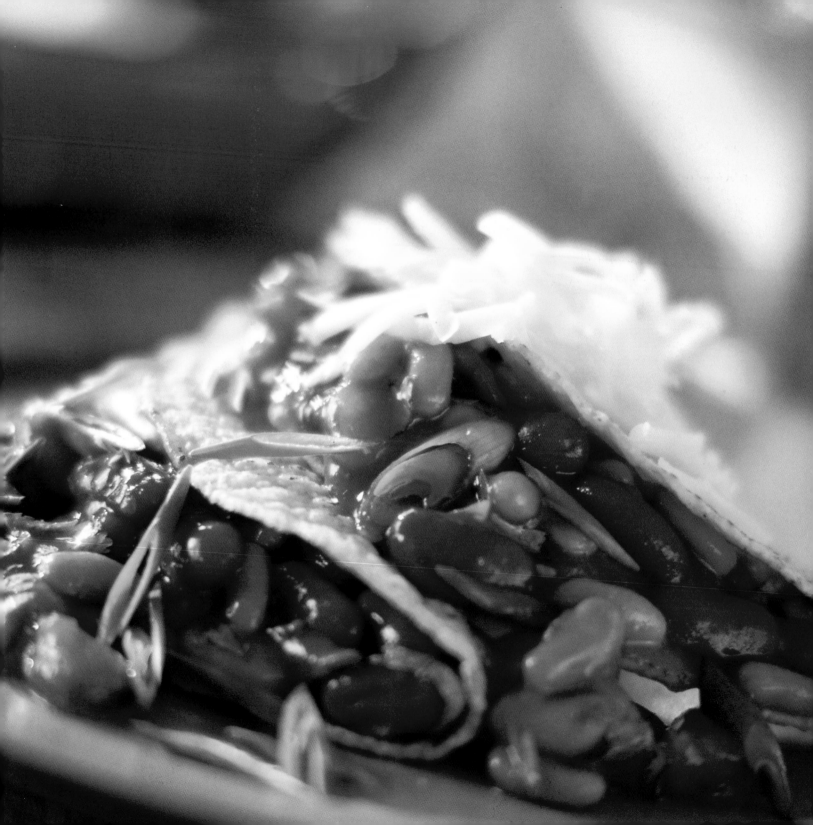

pineapple tarte tatin

This pineapple tart is a real treat, a delicious end to any meal. Almonds contain calcium, magnesium, boron, and essential fatty acids, all of which are good for healthy brain function and good memory.

▌ ingredients

- 5tbsp honey

- finely grated rind of 1 lemon

- 2 pounds (900g) pineapple, peeled, cored and sliced or chopped (approx 1¼ pounds (550g) prepared fruit)

- ¼ cup/1 ounce (25g) flaked almonds, toasted, to decorate

for the pastry

- 1½ cups/6 ounces (175g) whole-wheat flour

- ⅓ cup/3 ounces (85g) butter

- 2 tbsp/1 ounce (25g) sugar

- 1 medium egg yolk

serves *six*
preparation time *25 minutes*
cooking time *25–30 minutes*

▌ method

1 Preheat the oven to 400°F.
2 Lightly grease a shallow 9-inch (23cm) round nonstick cake pan and set aside.
3 Put the flour in a bowl, then lightly rub in the butter until the mixture resembles bread crumbs. Stir in the sugar, then add the egg yolk and enough cold water to make a soft dough. Set aside.
4 Warm the honey in a saucepan, then pour it over the bottom of the pan. Sprinkle the lemon rind over the honey. Arrange the pineapple decoratively in overlapping circles in the honey, covering the bottom completely.
5 Roll the dough out on a lightly floured surface to a round slightly larger than the pan. Lay the dough over the pineapple, tucking the excess dough down the edge.

6 Bake for 25–30 minutes, until the pastry is crisp and lightly browned.
7 Place a serving plate on top of the pan, invert, and remove the pan. Scatter the pineapple with flaked almonds.
8 Serve warm or cold in slices, with a little plain yogurt or crème fraîche.

variations

- *Use sliced eating apples or apricots instead of pineapple.*
- *Omit the lemon rind, if preferred.*
- *Use pineapple canned in fruit juice and drained, instead of fresh.*
- *Use the grated rind of 1 small orange instead of the lemon rind.*

desserts *and* bakes

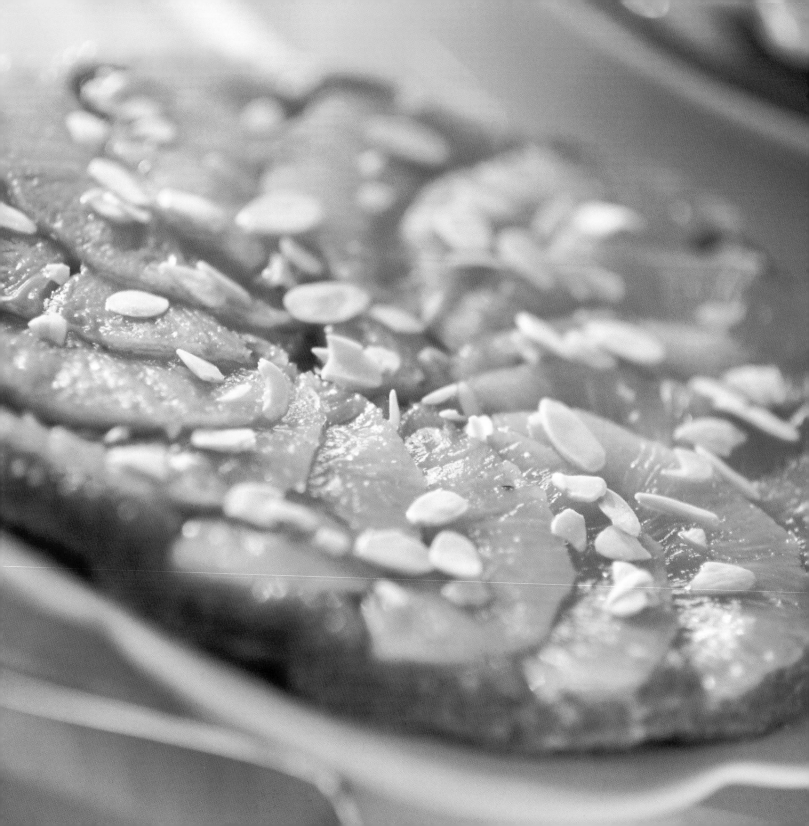

broiled fruit *with* yogurt

 Fresh fruits lightly broiled and served with plain yogurt make a quick and easy dessert. Yogurt contains substances that keep the brain alert.

ingredients

- 4 apricots
- 2 peaches
- 1 apple
- 1 pear
- 2 bananas
- 3tbsp honey
- 2tbsp unsweetened apple juice
- 1tbsp brandy
- 1–2tsp ground cinnamon
- yogurt, to serve

serves *four*
preparation time *15 minutes*
cooking time *4–6 minutes*

method

1 Dip the apricots and peaches in a large saucepan of boiling water for 15 seconds. Remove using a slotted spoon and plunge into a bowl of cold water. Drain, then peel off the skins.

2 Cover a broiler rack with foil. Preheat the broiler to high. Halve and pit the apricots, pit and thickly slice the peaches, and put them on the broiler rack.

3 Peel, core, and thinly slice the apple and pear. Peel and slice the bananas diagonally. Add to the other fruit on the broiler rack.

4 Put the honey, apple juice, brandy, and cinnamon in a small bowl and stir. Drizzle the mixture evenly over the fruit.

5 Broil the fruit for about 4–6 minutes, until hot or cooked as you like, turning once or twice.

6 Serve hot with some plain yogurt spooned alongside.

variations

- *Use maple syrup instead of honey.*
- *Use unsweetened orange juice or white grape juice instead of apple.*
- *Use rum instead of brandy.*
- *Use ground ginger or mixed spices instead of cinnamon.*

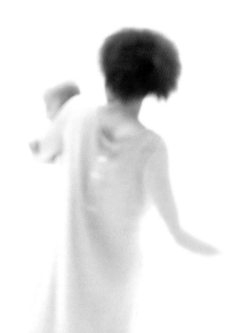

desserts *and* bakes

carrot *and* walnut cake

 This delicious cake is sure to be a favorite. Carrots and walnuts contain B vitamins, which are essential for mental alertness and memory.

■ ingredients

- ¾ cup/6 ounces (175g) softened butter
- ¾ cup/6 ounces (175g) light brown sugar
- 3 medium eggs, beaten
- 1½ cups/6 ounces (175g) whole-wheat flour
- ½ cup/2 ounces (55g) uncooked oatmeal
- 2tsp baking powder
- 2 cups/8 ounces (225g) grated carrots
- 1¼ cups/5 ounces (140g) chopped walnuts
- ⅔ cup/4 ounces (115g) golden raisins
- approx 2tbsp milk

for the topping

- 1 cup/8 ounces (225g) reduced fat cream cheese cheese
- 1–2tbsp honey
- 1tsp finely grated orange rind

serves *ten*
preparation time *20 minutes*
cooking time *1–1¼ hours*

■ method

1 Preheat the oven to 350°F.
2 Grease and line a deep, 8-inch (20cm) round cake pan.
3 Cream the butter and sugar together in a bowl until light and fluffy. Gradually beat in the eggs, beating well after each addition.
4 Fold in the flour, oatmeal, and baking powder, then fold in the carrots, 115g (4oz) walnuts, golden raisins, and a little milk to make a fairly soft dropping consistency.
5 Transfer the mixture to the cake pan and hollow the center slightly. bake for 1–1¼ hours until risen and firm to the touch.
6 Cool in the pan for a few minutes, then turn out onto a wire rack. Remove the lining paper and leave to cool completely.

7 To make the topping, fold the cream cheese, honey, and orange rind together, adding honey to taste. Spread over the top of the cold cake and sprinkle the remaining walnuts over the top.
8 Store the cake in the refrigerator until required.

variations

• *Omit the cream cheese topping and serve the cake plain.*
• *Use pecan nuts instead of walnuts.*
• *Use raisins or chopped dried apricots instead of golden raisins.*

freezing instructions

Let cool completely, then wrap in foil or seal in a freezer bag and label. Freeze for up to 3 months. Defrost for several hours at room temperature before serving.

desserts *and* bakes

you *must* remember this

PACKED FULL OF PROTEIN, *B group vitamins, as well as the minerals zinc, magnesium, boron, and selenium that are vital for brain function,* this unforgettable selection of nutritious recipes from the memory foods section can help to improve mental alertness and memory.

guacamole *with* vegetable crudités

Avocado is rich in the B vitamins—essential for brain function and quick recall.

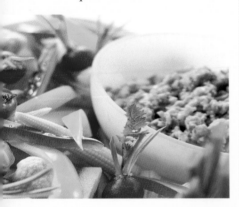

ingredients

- 2 ripe avocados
- juice of 1 small lime
- 3 shallots (French shallots), finely chopped
- 2 plum (Roma) tomatoes, peeled, seeded, and finely chopped
- 1 fresh green chili, seeded and finely chopped
- 1 clove garlic, crushed
- 1tbsp chopped fresh cilantro
- sea salt
- freshly ground black pepper
- fresh cilantro sprigs, to garnish
- prepared vegetable crudités, including carrot, cucumber and bell pepper sticks, baby corn, cauliflower florets, cherry tomatoes, and green onions

serves *four to six*
preparation time *10 minutes*

method

1 Peel and pit the avocados and put the flesh in a bowl. Mash the avocado flesh with the lime juice until smooth.
2 Stir in the shallots, tomatoes, chili, garlic, chopped cilantro, and seasoning.
3 Transfer the mixture to a serving dish. Garnish with fresh cilantro sprigs and serve immediately with a selection of raw vegetable crudités alongside.

chicken *and* garbanzo bean casserole

The garbanzo beans in this dish are a valuable source of zinc, not to mention the protein-rich chicken—both excellent brain nutrients.

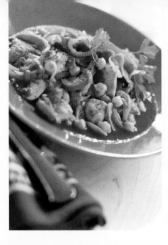

ingredients

- 1tbsp olive oil
- 1 pound (450g) skinless, boneless chicken breast, cut into 1-inch (2.5cm) cubes
- 8 ounces (225g) shallots (French shallots), sliced
- 2 leeks, washed and sliced
- 1 green bell pepper, seeded and diced
- 8 ounces (225g) mixed cremini and button mushrooms, sliced
- 1 cup/6 ounces (175g) frozen peas
- 2 14-ounce (400g) cans garbanzo beans, rinsed and drained
- 1 14-ounce (400g) can chopped tomatoes
- 1tbsp sun-dried tomato paste
- ²/₃ cup/¼ pint (150ml) chicken stock (see recipe on page 20)
- 1¼ cups/½ pint (300ml) dry white wine
- 1 bouquet garni
- sea salt and ground black pepper
- 1tbsp cornstarch (optional)
- fresh herb sprigs, to garnish

serves *six*
preparation time *25 minutes*
cooking time *1 hour*

method

1 Preheat the oven to 350°F.

2 Heat the oil in a large flameproof, ovenproof casserole. Add the chicken pieces and cook gently until lightly browned all over, stirring occasionally.

3 Stir in the shallots, leeks, green pepper, mushrooms, peas, and garbanzo beans.

4 Add the tomatoes, tomato paste, stock, wine, bouquet garni, and seasoning, and stir.

5 Bring to a boil, stirring occasionally then cover and bake for about 1 hour, until the chicken and vegetables are cooked and tender, stirring once or twice. Remove from the oven and discard the bouquet garni.

6 Blend the cornstarch, if using, with 3tbsp water and stir into the casserole. Heat gently, stirring continuously, until the mixture comes to a boil and thickens slightly. Simmer gently for 2 minutes, stirring occasionally.

7 Spoon onto warmed serving plates. Garnish with herb sprigs and serve with whole-wheat bread.

pineapple tarte tatin

Almonds make this dessert rich in calcium, magnesium, boron, and essential fatty acids—great for memory and brain function.

ingredients

- 5tbsp honey
- finely grated rind of 1 lemon
- 2 pounds (900g) pineapple, peeled, cored and sliced or chopped (approx 1¼ pounds (550g) prepared fruit)
- ¼ cup/1 ounce (25g) flaked almonds, toasted, to decorate

for the pastry

- 1½ cups/6 ounces (175g) whole-wheat flour
- ⅓ cup/3 ounces (85g) butter
- 2 tbsp/1 ounce (25g) sugar
- 1 medium egg yolk

serves *six*
preparation time *25 minutes*
cooking time *25–30 minutes*

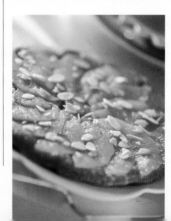

method

1 Preheat the oven to 400°F.

2 Lightly grease a shallow 9-inch (23cm) round nonstick cake pan and set aside.

3 Put the flour in a bowl, then lightly rub in the butter until the mixture resembles bread crumbs. Stir in the sugar, then add the egg yolk and enough cold water to make a soft dough. Set aside.

4 Warm the honey in a saucepan, then pour it over the bottom of the pan. Sprinkle the lemon rind over the honey. Arrange the pineapple decoratively in overlapping circles in the honey, covering the bottom completely.

5 Roll the dough out on a lightly floured surface to a round slightly larger than the pan. Lay the dough over the pineapple, tucking the excess dough down the edge.

6 Bake for 25–30 minutes, until the pastry is crisp and lightly browned.

7 Place a serving plate on top of the pan, invert, and remove the pan. Scatter the pineapple with flaked almonds.

8 Serve warm or cold in slices, with a little plain yogurt or crème fraîche.

focus *foods*

MINERALS ARE IMPORTANT *for healthy brain function. Zinc is needed for mental alertness and concentration—good sources are legumes, whole-grain bread and cereals, and fish. The trace element boron is needed in only tiny amounts but is essential for mental alertness. Boron is found in fresh and dried fruits, green vegetables, walnuts, almonds, and hazelnuts. A deficiency of iron may affect thinking in some people. Iron-rich foods include red meats, dark-meat poultry, organ meats, green leafy vegetables, nuts, dried fruits, whole grains, enriched breads and cereals, and fish.*

butternut squash *and* leek soup

 This mildly spiced soup is ideal for chilly days. Winter squash provides beta carotene, plus B vitamins and iron, essential for concentration.

ingredients

- 1 tbsp olive oil
- 1 onion, chopped
- 2 leeks, washed and thinly sliced
- 1 clove garlic, crushed
- 2 tsp ground coriander
- 2 tsp ground cumin
- 3½ cups/1 pound (450g) diced butternut squash—peeled and seeded weight
- 3½ cups/1½ pints (850ml vegetable stock (see recipe on page 20)
- sea salt
- freshly ground black pepper
- fresh herb sprigs, to garnish

serves *four*
preparation time *15 minutes*
cooking time *30 minutes*

method

1 Heat the oil in a large saucepan. Add the onion, leeks, and garlic, and cook gently for 3 minutes.
2 Add the ground spices and cook for 1 minute, stirring.
3 Stir in the squash, stock, and seasoning. Cover and bring to a boil; then reduce the heat and simmer for about 20 minutes, until the vegetables are cooked and tender, stirring occasionally.
4 Remove the pan from the heat and set aside to cool slightly; then purée the soup in a blender or food processor until smooth.
5 Return the soup to the rinsed-out saucepan and reheat until hot, stirring occasionally.
6 Ladle into warmed soup bowls to serve and garnish with fresh herb sprigs.
7 Serve with whole-wheat bread or toast.

variations

• *Use pumpkin flesh instead of butternut squash.*
• *Use 6 shallots (French shallots) instead of onion.*

freezing instructions

Let cool completely, then transfer to a rigid, freezeproof container. Cover, seal, and label. Freeze for up to 3 months. Defrost for several hours, or overnight in the refrigerator. Reheat gently in a saucepan until piping hot.

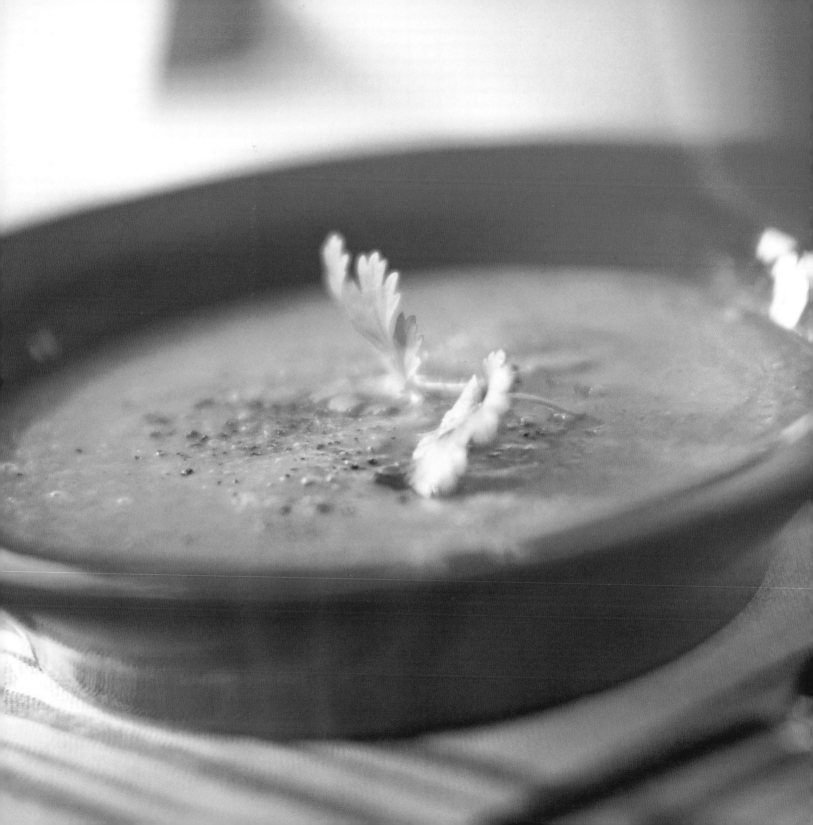

minted pea soup

A steaming hot bowl of homemade soup served with whole-wheat bread rolls makes an excellent appetizer for cold winter days. Peas are a good source of zinc, a nutrient needed by the brain for concentration.

ingredients

- 1tbsp olive oil
- 1 onion, chopped
- 2 leeks, washed and sliced
- 3 cups/1 pound (450g) fresh peas
- 3½ cups/1½ pints (850ml) vegetable stock (see recipe on page 20)
- sea salt
- freshly ground black pepper
- 2tbsp chopped fresh mint
- fresh mint sprigs, to garnish

serves *four*
preparation time *10 minutes*
cooking time *25–30 minutes*

method

1 Heat the oil in a large saucepan. Add the onion and leeks, and cook gently for 5 minutes, stirring.
2 Stir in the peas, stock, and seasoning. Cover and bring to a boil; then reduce the heat and simmer for 15–20 minutes, until the vegetables are tender.
3 Purée the soup in a food processor; then return it to the rinsed-out saucepan, add the chopped mint, and reheat.
4 Ladle into soup bowls and garnish with mint sprigs. Serve with whole-wheat rolls.

variations

• *Use frozen peas if fresh peas are not available.*
• *Use mushrooms or zucchini instead of peas.*

freezing instructions

Let cool completely, then transfer to a rigid, freezeproof container. Cover, seal, and label. Freeze for up to 3 months. Defrost for several hours, or overnight in the refrigerator. Reheat gently in a saucepan until piping hot.

tuna *and* garbanzo bean salad

Garbanzo beans, salad vegetables, and flaked tuna with a simple dressing make this a tasty appetizer. Fish contains the amino acid tyrosine, used to make brain-stimulating chemicals.

ingredients

- 1 14-ounce (400g) can garbanzo beans, rinsed and drained
- 8 ounces (225g) cherry tomatoes, halved
- 1 red bell pepper, seeded and diced
- half an English cucumber, diced
- 1 cup/4 ounces (115g) chopped sugar-snap peas (mangetout)
- 1 7-ounce (220g) can tuna in water, drained and flaked
- 4 ounces (115g) mixed salad leaves
- fresh herb sprigs, to garnish

for the dressing

- 4tbsp tomato juice
- 2tbsp olive oil
- 1tsp balsamic vinegar
- 1–2tbsp chopped fresh mixed herbs
- ½tsp sugar
- sea salt
- freshly ground black pepper

serves *six*
preparation time *15 minutes*

method

1 Put the garbanzo beans, cherry tomatoes, red pepper, cucumber, and sugar-snap peas (mangetout) in a bowl and mix well.
2 Put the tomato juice, olive oil, vinegar, chopped herbs, sugar, and seasoning in a small bowl and whisk together.
3 Pour the dressing over the vegetables and toss to mix. Add the flaked tuna and stir gently.
4 Arrange the mixed salad leaves on six serving plates and spoon some tuna mixture onto each plate. Garnish with herb sprigs.
5 Serve with crispbread or whole-wheat bread.

variations

• *Use canned salmon or crab instead of tuna.*
• *Use canned black-eyed peas or red kidney beans instead of garbanzo beans.*

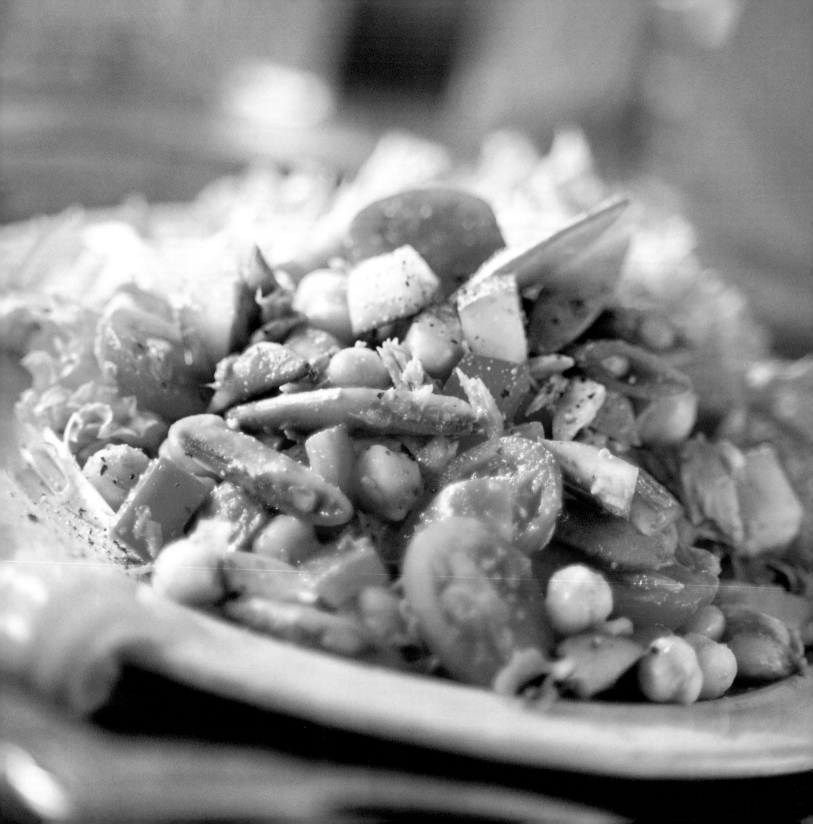

fettuccine *with* mussel sauce

 Freshly cooked pasta, topped with a generous serving of tomato and mussel sauce, makes a delicious meal. As a complex carbohydrate, pasta can help to calm an over-active mind and aids concentration.

ingredients

- I tbsp olive oil
- 4 shallots (French shallots) or I small onion, finely chopped
- I clove garlic, crushed
- I 14-ounce (400g) can chopped tomatoes
- 1¼ cups/¼ pint (150ml) dry white wine
- I tbsp tomato paste
- sea salt
- freshly ground black pepper
- 8 ounces (225g) fettuccine
- 8 ounces (225g) cooked, shelled small mussels
- 2 tbsp chopped fresh flat-leaf parsley
- 6–8 cooked fresh mussels in their shells
- fresh flat-leaf parsley sprigs, to garnish

serves *two*
preparation time *10 minutes*
cooking time *25 minutes*

method

I Heat the oil in a saucepan and add the shallots or onion and garlic. Cook for 5 minutes, stirring occasionally, until soft.

2 Stir in the tomatoes, wine, tomato paste, and seasoning. Bring to a boil, then simmer, uncovered, for about 15 minutes, until the sauce has thickened, stirring occasionally.

3 Meanwhile, cook the pasta in a large saucepan of lightly salted, boiling water for 10–12 minutes, until just cooked or *al dente*.

4 Stir the mussels and chopped parsley into the tomato sauce and cook for about 5 minutes, until piping hot.

5 Drain the pasta thoroughly and place onto warmed serving plates. Spoon the mussel sauce over the pasta and garnish with mussels in their shells and the parsley sprigs.

6 Serve hot with a mixed dark-green leaf side salad.

variations

- *Use spaghetti or tagliatelle instead of fettuccine.*
- *Use cooked, shelled shrimp instead of mussels.*
- *Use red wine instead of white wine.*
- *Add I finely chopped, seeded fresh red chili to the sauce with the tomatoes.*

fish *dishes*

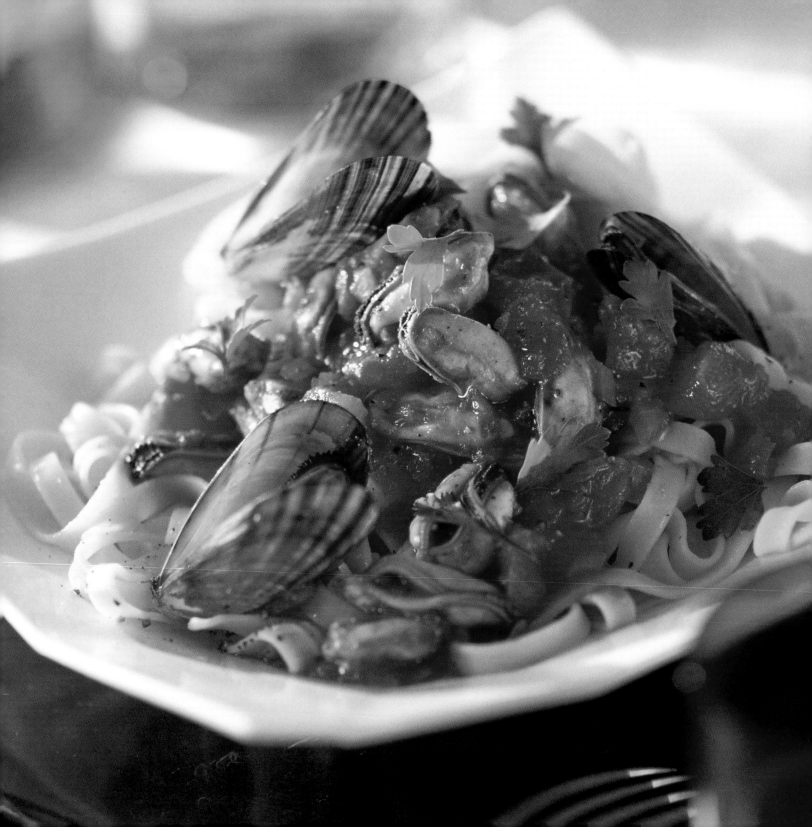

baked stuffed trout

Baked stuffed trout is delicious served with cooked fresh vegetables. Oily fish such as trout provide essential fatty acids, and enriched oatmeal provides iron, both important nutrients for healthy brain tissue and good concentration.

ingredients

- I tbsp olive oil
- I small onion, finely chopped
- I cup/3 ounces (85g) finely chopped fresh shiitake or oyster mushrooms
- ⅓ cup/I ounce (25g) uncooked oatmeal
- ¼ cup/I ounce (25g) finely chopped hazelnuts or almonds
- finely grated rind of I small lemon
- I tbsp chopped fresh parsley
- sea salt
- freshly ground black pepper
- 4 rainbow trout, each weighing about 10 ounces (280g), gutted and cleaned, with heads and tails left on
- juice of 2 lemons
- fresh parsley sprigs, to garnish

serves *four*
preparation time *20 minutes*
cooking time *30–40 minutes*

method

I Preheat the oven to 350°F.
2 Heat the oil in a saucepan. Add the onion and mushrooms and cook for about 5 minutes, until softened, stirring occasionally.
3 Remove the pan from the heat and add the oatmeal, hazelnuts or almonds, lemon rind, chopped parsley, and seasoning; mix well. Spoon some of the oatmeal mixture into each trout.
4 Place the trout side-by-side in a shallow, ovenproof dish and drizzle the lemon juice over the fish.
5 Cover with foil and bake for 30–40 minutes, until the fish is cooked and the flesh flakes when tested with a fork.
6 Garnish with fresh parsley sprigs and serve with cooked fresh vegetables such as new potatoes, green cabbage, and carrots.

variations

- *Use mackerel instead of trout.*
- *Use button mushrooms instead of shiitake or oyster mushrooms.*
- *Use Brazil nuts or walnuts instead of hazelnuts or almonds.*

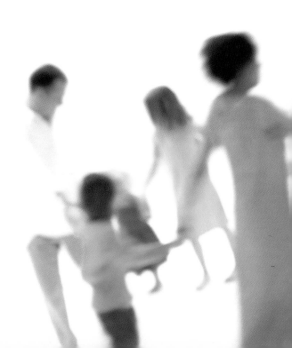

fish *dishes*

chicken, tomato, *and* red wine casserole

This delicious chicken casserole, served with mashed potatoes and cooked fresh vegetables, is a popular family dish. As a high-protein food, chicken is good for stimulating the brain and increasing the ability to focus.

ingredients

- 1tbsp olive oil
- 4 skinless chicken portions (2 leg and 2 breast portions)
- 12 ounces (350g) pearl onions
- 4 carrots, sliced
- 2 celery stalks, chopped
- 12 ounces (350g) baby button mushrooms
- 1 clove garlic, crushed
- 1 14-ounce (400g) can chopped tomatoes
- 1¼ cups/½ pint (300ml) red wine
- ⅔ cup/¼ pint (150ml) chicken stock (see recipe on page 20)
- 2tsp dried *herbes de provence*
- sea salt
- freshly ground black pepper
- 2tbsp cornstarch
- fresh herb sprigs, to garnish

serves *four*
preparation time *15 minutes*
cooking time *1½ hours*

method

1 Preheat the oven to 350°F.
2 Heat the oil in a large flameproof, ovenproof casserole dish. Add the chicken and cook gently until sealed all over, turning once or twice.
3 Remove the dish from the heat and stir in the onions, carrots, celery, mushrooms, garlic, tomatoes, wine, stock, dried herbs, and seasoning.
4 Cover and bake for about 1½ hours, until the chicken and vegetables are cooked and tender, stirring once or twice.
5 Remove from the oven. Using a slotted spoon, remove the chicken from the casserole and place on a warmed plate; cover and keep hot.
6 Blend the cornstarch with 4tbsp water and stir into the casserole. Bring to a boil, stirring continuously, until the vegetable sauce thickens slightly. Simmer gently for 2 minutes, stirring.

7 Place the chicken portions on warmed serving plates and spoon some vegetable sauce over. Garnish with the herb sprigs.
8 Serve with mashed potatoes, green beans, and parsnips.

variations

- *Use white wine or medium cider instead of red wine.*
- *Use shallots (French shallots) instead of pearl onions.*
- *Use parsnips instead of carrots.*

freezing instructions

Let cool completely, then transfer to a rigid, freezeproof container. Cover, seal, and label. Freeze for up to 3 months. Defrost for several hours, or overnight in the refrigerator. Reheat in a moderate oven until piping hot.

turkey *with* herbed mustard sauce

Pan-fried turkey breast steaks served with a mild mustard sauce make a tempting dish for a main meal. Turkey is a good source of B vitamins, selenium, protein, and zinc, all of which are essential to brain function.

ingredients

- I tbsp olive oil
- I tbsp/½ ounce (15g) butter
- 4 turkey breasts, each weighing about 4½ ounces (125g)

for the sauce

- 2tbsp cornstarch
- ¾ cup/7 fluid ounces (200ml) milk
- ⅔ cup/½ pint (150ml) vegetable stock, cooled (see recipe on page 20)
- I tbsp whole-grain mustard
- I tsp mixed dried herbs
- I tsp honey
- sea salt
- freshly ground black pepper
- fresh herb sprigs, to garnish

serves *four*
preparation time *10 minutes*
cooking time *20 minutes*

method

1 Heat the oil and butter gently in a non-stick skillet until the butter is melted. Add the turkey breasts and cook gently for about 20 minutes, turning once, until cooked, tender, and lightly browned all over.

2 Meanwhile, make the mustard sauce. In a saucepan, blend the cornstarch with a little of the milk. Stir in the remaining milk and stock, then heat gently, stirring continuously, until the sauce comes to a boil and thickens. Simmer gently for 2 minutes, stirring.

3 Stir in the mustard, dried herbs, honey, and seasoning, and heat gently until piping hot, stirring.

4 Serve the turkey breasts with the mustard sauce poured over. Garnish with herb sprigs.

5 Serve with baked potatoes, broiled bell peppers, and eggplants or zucchini.

variations

• *Use chicken breast portions instead of turkey.*

• *Use I tbsp chopped fresh mixed herbs instead of dried herbs.*

• *Add an extra I tbsp whole-grain mustard to the sauce for a stronger mustard flavor.*

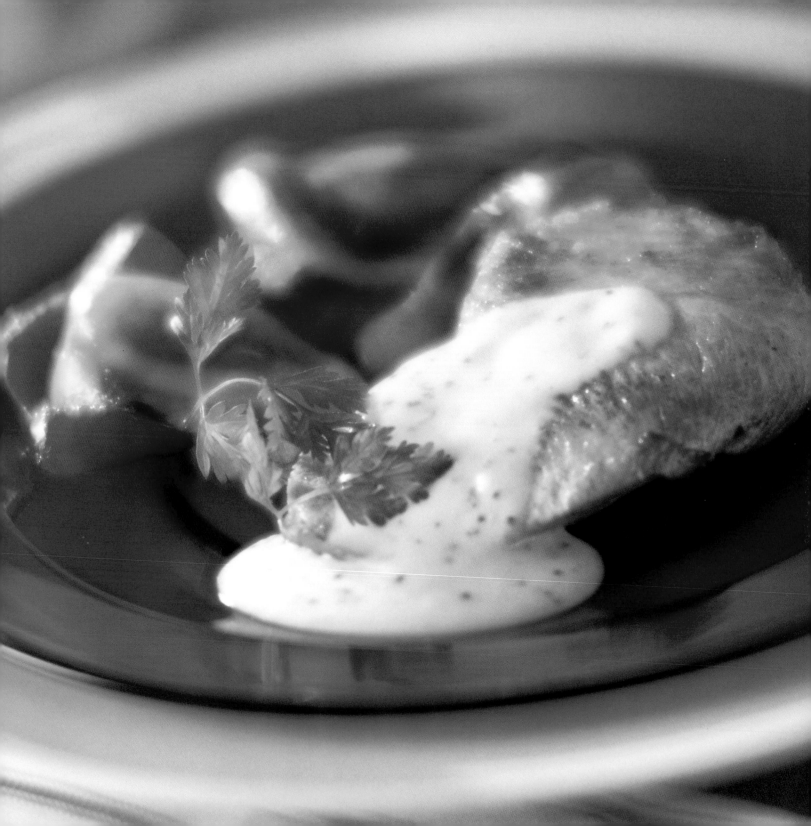

ratatouille *and* bean pot

 The addition of beans to ratatouille adds flavor and texture. Beans are an excellent source of iron, which is an essential nutrient for brain function.

ingredients

- 2 onions, sliced
- 2 cloves garlic, thinly sliced
- 1 eggplant, sliced
- 2 zucchini, sliced
- 1 each green, red, and yellow bell pepper, seeded and sliced
- 1 14-ounce (400g) can chopped tomatoes
- 6tbsp red wine
- 1tbsp tomato paste
- 2tsp dried *herbes de provence*
- 1 14-ounce (400g) can red kidney beans, rinsed and drained
- 1 14 ounce (400g) can black-eyed peas, rinsed and drained
- sea salt
- freshly ground black pepper
- fresh herb sprigs, to garnish

serves *four to six*
preparation time *15 minutes*
cooking time *1 hour*

method

1 Preheat the oven to 350°F.
2 Put all the ingredients, except the herb garnish, in a large ovenproof casserole and mix well. Cover and bake for about 1 hour, until the vegetables are cooked and tender, stirring once or twice.
3 Garnish with the herb sprigs and serve hot or cold with crusty whole-wheat bread or baked potatoes topped with a little grated Cheddar cheese.

variations

• *Use unsweetened apple juice or medium cider instead of red wine.*
• *Use canned garbanzo beans and green beans instead of red kidney beans and black-eyed peas.*
• *Add 8 ounces (225g) baby button mushrooms to the vegetable mixture before cooking.*

freezing instructions

Let cool completely, then transfer to a rigid, freezeproof container. Cover, seal, and label. Freeze for up to 3 months. Defrost for several hours, or overnight in the refrigerator. Reheat gently in a saucepan or in a moderate oven until piping hot.

vegetable *dishes*

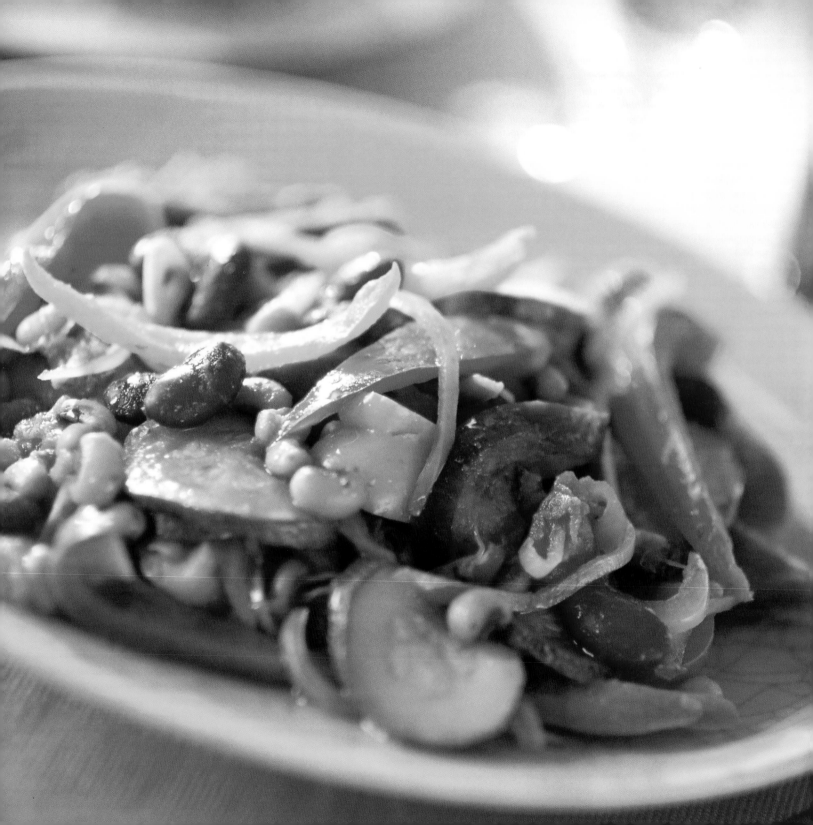

roast new potatoes *with* shallots

 This is a delicious way of serving new potatoes. Potatoes are a complex carbohydrate, good for helping you to focus and concentrate.

ingredients

- 1 pound (450g) baby new potatoes
- 12 ounces (350g) small shallots (French shallots)
- 2tbsp olive oil
- sea salt
- freshly ground black pepper
- 1tbsp chopped fresh parsley (optional)
- 1tbsp chopped fresh mint (optional)
- fresh mint sprigs, to garnish

serves *four* *as an accompaniment*
preparation time *10 minutes*
cooking time *45–60 minutes*

method

1 Preheat the oven to 400°F.
2 Put the potatoes and shallots in a roasting pan. Add the oil and seasoning, and toss until the vegetables are coated all over.
3 Bake for 45–60 minutes, until the vegetables are cooked, tender, and golden brown, stirring once or twice.
4 Sprinkle over the chopped herbs, if using, and stir. Garnish with the mint sprigs and serve with cooked fresh vegetables such as chopped spinach and carrots.

variations

• *Use pearl onions instead of shallots.*
• *Use sesame oil instead of olive oil.*
• *Use chopped fresh mixed herbs instead of the parsley and mint.*

okra *with* spicy tomato sauce

This dish makes a great accompaniment to broiled chicken or fish. Tomatoes provide vitamin C, a nutrient good for a healthy brain.

ingredients

- 1½ pounds (700g) peeled, seeded, and chopped tomatoes
- 6 shallots (French shallots), thinly sliced
- 1 small leek, washed and thinly sliced
- 2 celery stalks, finely chopped
- 1 clove garlic, crushed
- ⅔ cup/¼ pint (150ml) red wine
- 2tbsp sun-dried tomato paste
- 2tsp ground cumin
- 1tsp ground coriander
- 1tsp hot chili powder
- sea salt
- freshly ground black pepper
- 1½ pounds (700g) okra

serves *six*
preparation time *15 minutes*
cooking time *25 minutes*

method

1 Put the tomatoes, shallots, leek, celery, garlic, wine, tomato paste, ground spices, and seasoning in a saucepan and mix well.
2 Bring to a boil; then reduce the heat, cover, and simmer for about 25 minutes, until the vegetables are tender.
3 Purée the vegetables in a food processor; then return to the rinsed-out saucepan and reheat.
4 Cook the okra in boiling water for about 5 minutes, until tender.
5 Serve the okra with the tomato sauce spooned over, with whole-wheat rolls, baked potatoes, or brown rice.

variations

• *Serve the spicy tomato sauce with other cooked fresh vegetables such as baby corn or baby zucchini.*
• *Use 1 onion instead of shallots.*
• *Use unsweetened apple juice or white wine instead of red wine.*

vegetable dishes

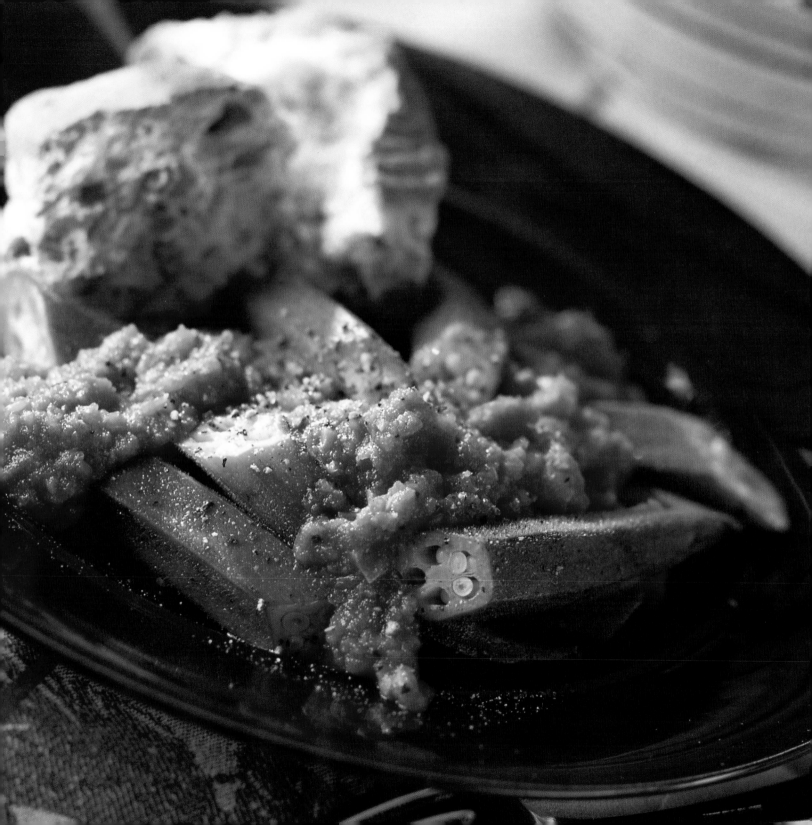

chocolate, apple, *and* raisin cake

This delicious fruity chocolate cake also makes an ideal dessert served with homemade custard or plain yogurt. Dried fruit such as golden raisins provides iron, magnesium, and B vitamins, all good for a healthy brain and nervous system.

■ ingredients

- ¾ cup/6 ounces (175g) softened butter
- ¾ cup/6 ounces (175g) light brown sugar
- 3 medium eggs, beaten
- 2½ cups/10 ounces (280g) plain whole-wheat flour
- 2tsp baking powder
- 1tsp ground mixed spices or cinnamon
- 3tbsp cocoa powder, sifted
- 2½ cups/12 ounces (350g) peeled, cored, and diced cooking apples
- 1 cup/6 ounces (175g) golden raisins
- approx 6tbsp milk
- 6 squares/6 ounces (175g) dark chocolate, roughly chopped

serves *ten*
preparation time *20 minutes*
cooking time *1¼–1½ hours*

■ method

1 Preheat the oven to 325°F.
2 Grease and line a deep 8-inch (20cm) round cake pan.
3 Cream the butter and sugar in a bowl until light and fluffy. Gradually beat in the eggs, beating well after each addition.
4 Fold in the flour, baking powder, mixed spices, and cocoa powder; then fold in the apples, golden raisins, and enough milk to give a fairly soft dropping consistency. Fold in the chocolate.
5 Transfer the mixture to the cake pan and level the surface. Bake for 1¼–1½ hours, until risen and firm to the touch.
6 Cool in the pan for a few minutes, then turn out onto a wire rack. Remove the lining paper and leave to cool completely.
7 Serve the apple cake warm or cold with a little homemade custard, plain yogurt, crème fraîche, or light sour cream.

variations

• Use chopped dried dates or chopped ready-to-eat dried apricots instead of golden raisins.
• Brush the cake with a little warmed honey or maple syrup and sprinkle with cane sugar just before serving.

freezing instructions

Let cool completely, then wrap in foil or seal in a freezer bag and label. Freeze for up to 3 months. Defrost for several hours at room temperature before serving.

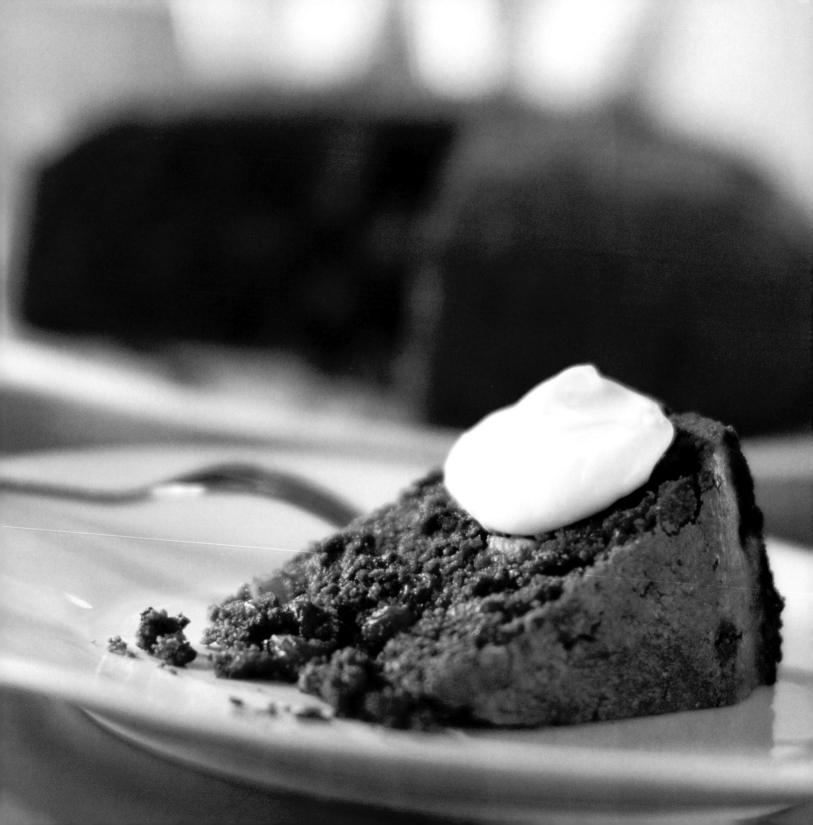

compote *of* winter fruits

Fresh winter fruits soaked in a fruit juice mixture are delicious served with a little plain yogurt, crème fraîche, or light sour cream. Fresh fruit is a good source of vitamin C, a nutrient that helps with the absorption of iron, and both are important nutrients for good brain function.

ingredients

- ¾ cup/7 fl oz (200ml) unsweetened apple juice
- ¾ cup/7 fl oz (200ml) unsweetened white grape juice
- 2tbsp ginger wine or ginger ale
- 2 cinnamon sticks, broken in half
- 6 whole cloves
- 1 baby pineapple
- 1 ripe medium mango
- 1 star fruit (carambola)
- 6 ounces (175g) fresh dates
- 1 apple
- 1 pear
- 2 kiwi fruit
- fresh mint sprigs, to decorate

serves *six*
preparation time *15 minutes*
cooking time *10 minutes*

method

1 Put the fruit juices, ginger wine, cinnamon sticks, and cloves, in a saucepan and heat gently until boiling. Remove from the heat.
2 Meanwhile, prepare the fruit. Peel, core, and chop the pineapple. Peel, pit, and dice the mango. Slice the star fruit (carambola). Pit and chop the dates. Peel, core, and slice the apple and pear. Peel and slice the kiwi fruit. Put the prepared fruit in a serving bowl and stir.
3 Pour the hot fruit juice mixture over the fruit and stir gently. Set aside to cool; then cover and chill before serving.
4 Remove and discard the cinnamon sticks and cloves before serving. Decorate with fresh mint sprigs and serve with plain yogurt, crème fraîche, or light sour cream.

variations

- *Use unsweetened orange juice and pineapple juice instead of the apple and grape juices.*
- *Use a melon instead of pineapple.*
- *Use brandy, rum, or fruit liqueur instead of ginger wine.*

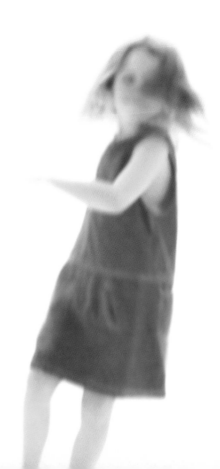

desserts *and* bakes

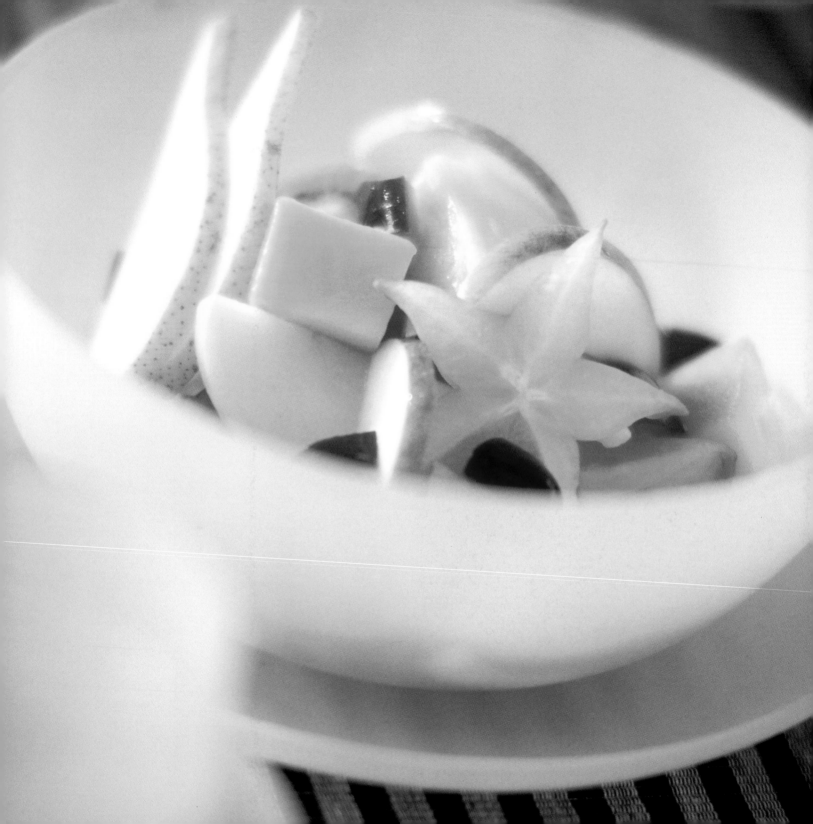

quiz *night*

B E QUICK OFF THE *mark on quiz night—this selection of recipes from the focus foods section provides excellent nourishment for your brain* and enhances the ability to focus, as the recipes contain the B-group vitamins as well as other essential nutrients such as zinc, boron, and iron.

tuna *and* garbanzo bean salad

An excellent source of the amino acid tyrosine, the tuna in this recipe will aid concentration.

ingredients

- 1 14-ounce (400g) can garbanzo beans, rinsed and drained
- 8 ounces (225g) cherry tomatoes, halved
- 1 red bell pepper, seeded and diced
- half an English cucumber, diced
- 1 cup/4 ounces (115g) chopped sugar-snap peas (mangetout)
- 1 7-ounce (220g) can tuna in water, drained and flaked
- 4 ounces (115g) mixed salad leaves
- fresh herb sprigs, to garnish

for the dressing

- 4tbsp tomato juice
- 2tbsp olive oil
- 1tsp balsamic vinegar
- 1–2tbsp chopped fresh mixed herbs
- ½tsp sugar
- sea salt
- freshly ground black pepper

serves *six*
preparation time *15 minutes*

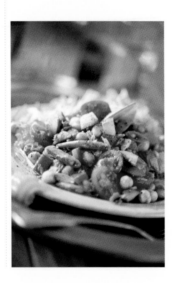

method

1 Put the garbanzo beans, cherry tomatoes, red pepper, cucumber, and sugar-snap peas (mangetout) in a bowl and mix well.
2 Put the tomato juice, olive oil, vinegar, chopped herbs, sugar, and seasoning in a small bowl and whisk together.
3 Pour the dressing over the vegetables and toss to mix. Add the flaked tuna and stir gently.
4 Arrange the mixed salad leaves on six serving plates and spoon some tuna mixture onto each plate. Garnish with herb sprigs.
5 Serve with crispbread or whole-wheat bread.

turkey *with* herbed mustard sauce

A succulent all-around winner when it comes to focusing the mind, turkey contains B vitamins, selenium, protein, and zinc.

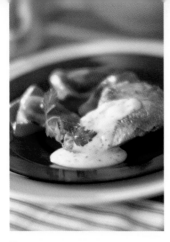

ingredients

- 1 tbsp olive oil
- 1 tbsp/½ ounce (15g) butter
- 4 turkey breasts, each weighing about 4½ ounces (125g)

for the sauce

- 2 tbsp cornstarch
- ¾ cup/7 fluid ounces (200ml) milk
- ⅔ cup/½ pint (150ml) vegetable stock, cooled (see recipe on page 20)
- 1 tbsp whole-grain mustard
- 1 tsp mixed dried herbs
- 1 tsp honey
- sea salt
- freshly ground black pepper
- fresh herb sprigs, to garnish

serves *four*
preparation time *10 minutes*
cooking time *20 minutes*

method

1 Heat the oil and butter gently in a non-stick skillet until the butter is melted. Add the turkey breasts and cook gently for about 20 minutes, turning once, until cooked, tender, and lightly browned all over.
2 Meanwhile, make the mustard sauce. In a saucepan, blend the cornstarch with a little of the milk. Stir in the remaining milk and stock, then heat gently, stirring continuously, until the sauce comes to a boil and thickens. Simmer gently for 2 minutes, stirring.
3 Stir in the mustard, dried herbs, honey, and seasoning, and heat gently until piping hot, stirring.
4 Serve the turkey breasts with the mustard sauce poured over. Garnish with herb sprigs.
5 Serve with baked potatoes, broiled bell peppers, and eggplants or zucchini.

compote *of* winter fruits

A juicy way to round off this mind-strengthening menu—most fresh fruits provide plenty of vitamin C.

ingredients

- ¾ cup/7 fl oz (200ml) unsweetened apple juice
- ¾ cup/7 fl oz (200ml) unsweetened white grape juice
- 2 tbsp ginger wine or ginger ale
- 2 cinnamon sticks, broken in half
- 6 whole cloves
- 1 baby pineapple
- 1 ripe medium mango
- 1 star fruit (carambola)
- 6 ounces (175g) fresh dates
- 1 apple
- 1 pear
- 2 kiwi fruit
- fresh mint sprigs, to decorate

serves *six*
preparation time *15 minutes*
cooking time *10 minutes*

method

1 Put the fruit juices, ginger wine, cinnamon sticks, and cloves, in a saucepan and heat gently until boiling. Remove from the heat.
2 Meanwhile, prepare the fruit. Peel, core, and chop the pineapple. Peel, pit, and dice the mango. Slice the star fruit (carambola). Pit and chop the dates. Peel, core, and slice the apple and pear. Peel and slice the kiwi fruit. Put the prepared fruit in a serving bowl and stir.
3 Pour the hot fruit juice mixture over the fruit and stir gently. Set aside to cool; then cover and chill before serving.
4 Remove and discard the cinnamon sticks and cloves before serving. Decorate with fresh mint sprigs and serve with plain yogurt, crème fraîche, or light sour cream.

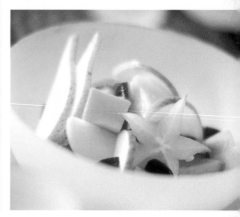

mental energy *foods*

PROTEIN FOODS CONTAIN *amino acids that stimulate the brain and so encourage clear thinking. If you have a demanding day's work ahead of you, eat scrambled eggs or yogurt and other dairy products for breakfast. Fish, chicken, lean meats, and legumes are also excellent sources of protein. Note that protein foods eaten at night may over-activate the brain and keep you awake.*

Fish and shellfish contain an amino acid called tyrosine, used to make the brain-stimulating chemicals noradrenalin and dopamine, which increase mental energy and alertness.

warm chicken salad *with* mango

This appetizing salad combines different textures and flavors. Cold-pressed oils and walnuts contain essential fatty acids needed by every cell in the body. They are especially important for healthy brain tissue and mental alertness.

ingredients

- 2 ounces (55g) baby spinach leaves
- 2 ounces (55g) watercress
- 6 ounces (175g) cherry tomatoes, halved
- 1 ripe medium mango, peeled, pitted, and diced
- 6–8 green onions, chopped
- ½ cup/2 ounces (55g) roughly chopped, pitted black olives
- ½ cup/2 ounces (55g) roughly chopped walnuts
- 1 tbsp olive oil
- 8 ounces (225g) skinless, boneless chicken breast, cut into thin strips
- fresh herb sprigs, to garnish

for the dressing

- 2 tbsp walnut oil
- 1 tbsp olive oil
- 1 tbsp red wine vinegar
- sea salt
- freshly ground black pepper

serves *four*
preparation time *15 minutes*
cooking time *5–7 minutes*

method

1 Put the spinach leaves, watercress, cherry tomatoes, mango, green onions, olives, and walnuts in a bowl and toss together. Divide the salad among four serving plates.

2 Put the walnut oil, 1 tbsp olive oil, vinegar, and seasoning in a small bowl and whisk until thoroughly mixed. Set aside.
3 Heat the remaining olive oil in a nonstick wok or large skillet. Add the chicken and stir-fry over a medium heat for about 5–7 minutes, until cooked, tender, and lightly browned all over.
4 Top each salad with some hot chicken. Give the dressing a quick whisk, then drizzle a little dressing over each salad.
5 Garnish with the herb sprigs and serve with crispbread or whole-wheat bread.

variations

- *Use skinless turkey breast or lean beef or lamb instead of chicken.*
- *Use 1 ripe avocado, peeled, pitted, diced, and tossed in a little lemon juice instead of the mango.*
- *Use pecan nuts or hazelnuts instead of walnuts.*
- *Use hazelnut oil or olive oil instead of walnut oil.*

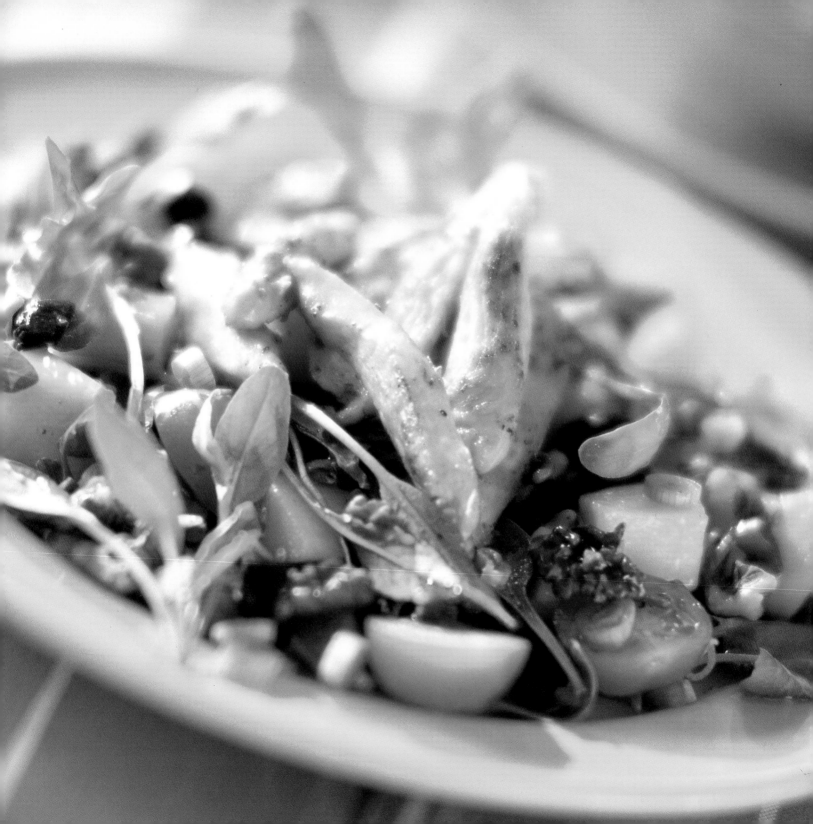

creamy carrot *and* celeriac soup

This creamy soup is a delicious appetizer or snack. Carrots contain beta carotene, an important antioxidant. Fresh culinary herbs such as cilantro make this dish even more nutritious.

ingredients

- 2 tbsp/1 ounce (25g) butter
- 1 large onion, chopped
- 12 ounces (350g) carrots, sliced
- 2½ cups/12 ounces (350g) diced celeriac
- 2½ cups/1 pint (600ml) vegetable stock (see recipe on page 20)
- sea salt
- freshly ground black pepper
- 1¼ cups/½ pint (300ml) milk
- 1–2tbsp chopped fresh cilantro (optional)
- fresh cilantro sprigs, to garnish

serves *four*
preparation time *15 minutes*
cooking time *40–45 minutes*

method

1 Melt the butter in a large saucepan. Add the onion, carrots and celeriac and cook gently for 5 minutes, stirring occasionally.
2 Add the stock and seasoning, and stir. Cover and bring to a boil; then reduce the heat and simmer for 30–40 minutes, until the vegetables are cooked and tender, stirring occasionally.
3 Remove the pan from the heat and set aside to cool slightly; then purée the soup in a blender or food processor until smooth.
4 Return the soup to the rinsed-out saucepan. Add the milk and chopped cilantro, if using, and reheat gently until piping hot, stirring occasionally.
5 Ladle into warmed soup bowls to serve and garnish with fresh cilantro sprigs.
6 Serve with warm fresh whole-wheat bread rolls.

variations

- Use parsnips instead of celeriac.
- Use rutabaga instead of carrots.
- Use chopped fresh mixed herbs or parsley instead of cilantro.

freezing instructions

Let cool completely, then transfer to a rigid, freezeproof container. Cover, seal, and label. Freeze for up to 3 months. Defrost for several hours, or overnight in the refrigerator. Reheat gently in a saucepan until piping hot.

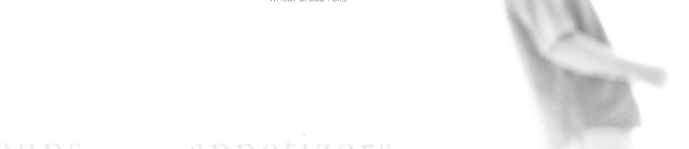

soups appetizers

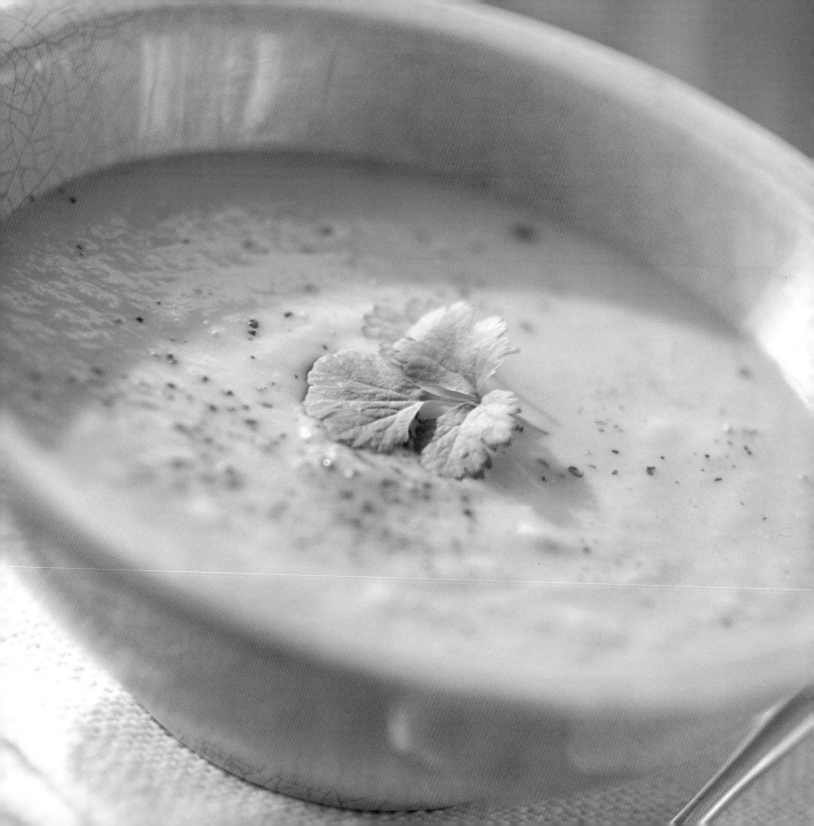

lemon sole *with* wild mushrooms

Broiled lemon sole fillets are delicious served with a wild mushroom sauce. Fish contains an amino acid used to make brain-stimulating chemicals that increase mental energy and alertness.

ingredients

- 2 tbsp/1 ounce (25g) butter
- 2 shallots (French shallots), thinly sliced
- 1 clove garlic, crushed
- 12 ounces/350g mixed fresh wild (field) mushrooms, such as shiitake and oyster mushrooms, sliced
- 2tbsp dry sherry
- 2–3tsp chopped fresh thyme (optional)
- sea salt
- freshly ground black pepper
- 2tbsp crème fraîche or light sour cream
- 8 lemon sole fillets
- a little olive oil, for brushing
- fresh thyme sprigs, to garnish

serves *four*
preparation time *10 minutes*
cooking time *10–15 minutes*

method

1 Preheat the broiler to medium. Line a broiler rack with foil.
2 Melt the butter in a large non-stick skillet. Add the shallots and garlic, and cook gently for 3 minutes, stirring occasionally.
3 Add the mushrooms and cook for about 5 minutes until tender, stirring occasionally.
4 Stir in the sherry, chopped thyme, if using, and seasoning. Increase the heat slightly and cook for 2–3 minutes, stirring until most of the liquid has evaporated.
5 Stir in the crème fraîche and adjust the seasoning.
6 Meanwhile, cook the fish. Place the lemon sole on the broiler rack and brush them lightly all over with oil. Broil for 4–6 minutes, until the fish is cooked and the flesh just flakes when tested with a fork, carefully turning over once during cooking.

7 Place two cooked fish fillets on each warmed serving plate and spoon some mushroom sauce on top or alongside. Garnish with fresh thyme sprigs and serve with sautéed potatoes, cooked green cabbage, and baby corn.

variations

- *Use firm white fish steaks instead of lemon sole and increase the cooking time a little.*
- *Use button or chestnut mushrooms instead of wild ones.*
- *Use brandy instead of sherry.*
- *Use chopped fresh sage or tarragon instead of thyme.*

fish

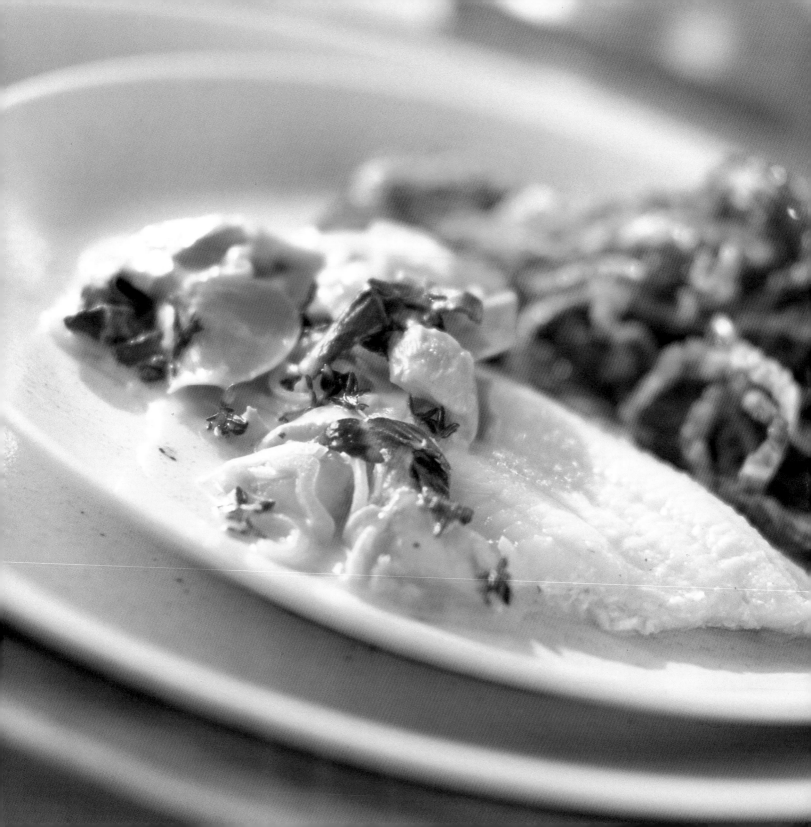

shrimp pasta salad

In this tasty dish, cooked pasta, vegetables, shrimp, and avocado are tossed together in a mayonnaise dressing. Shrimp contain the mineral zinc, which is necessary for a healthy brain and nervous system.

ingredients

- 8 ounces (225g) pasta twists (spirals)
- 8 ounces (225g) small broccoli florets
- 8tbsp mayonnaise (see recipe on page 21)
- 2tbsp chopped fresh chives
- 1tsp finely grated lemon rind
- sea salt
- freshly ground black pepper
- ½ cup/2 ounces (55g) shredded round lettuce
- ½ cup/2 ounces (25g) chopped watercress
- 8 ounces (225g) cooked, shelled shrimp
- 1 ripe avocado
- 1tbsp fresh lemon juice
- fresh chive, to garnish

serves *four to six*
preparation time *10 minutes*
cooking time *10 minutes*

method

1 Cook the pasta in a large saucepan of lightly salted, boiling water for 8–10 minutes, until just cooked or *al dente*. Drain, rinse under cold running water, and drain thoroughly again. Set aside to cool completely.
2 Blanch the broccoli in a saucepan of boiling water for 3 minutes. Cool under cold running water; then drain thoroughly and set aside.
3 Put the cold pasta in a large bowl. In a small bowl, mix the mayonnaise, chopped chives, lemon rind, and seasoning. Add to the pasta and stir.
4 Stir in the broccoli, lettuce, watercress, and shrimp. Peel, pit, and dice the avocado and toss with the lemon juice. Add to the pasta salad and stir gently.
5 Serve immediately, or cover and chill before serving.
6 Garnish with the chives and serve with crusty whole-wheat bread rolls.

variations

- *Use chopped fresh basil or parsley instead of chives.*
- *Use finely grated lime or orange rind instead of lemon rind.*
- *Use canned flaked tuna or salmon instead of shrimp.*

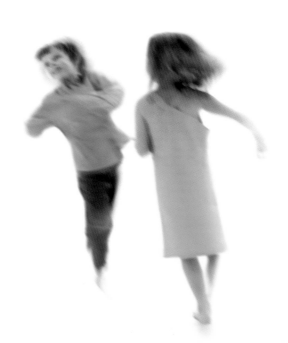

fish

lamb brochettes *with* herbed rice

 Succulent lean lamb grilled with mixed vegetables make tasty kebabs. Lamb is packed with protein for healthy brain function.

ingredients

- 8 ounces (225g) long-grain brown rice
- 12 small shallots (French shallots)
- 12 baby corn
- 12 ounces (350g) lean lamb, cut into 1-inch (2.5cm) cubes
- 2 small red bell peppers, each cut into 8 pieces
- 1 zucchini, cut into 16 thin slices
- 8 bay leaves
- 6tbsp red wine
- 2tbsp olive oil
- 2tsp mustard
- 1 clove garlic, crushed
- sea salt
- freshly ground black pepper
- 2–3tbsp chopped fresh mixed herbs

serves *four*
preparation time *15 minutes*
cooking time *35 minutes*

method

1 Cook the rice in a large saucepan of lightly salted, boiling water for about 35 minutes, until cooked and tender. Drain well and rinse with hot water; drain again and keep hot.
2 Meanwhile, cook the shallots and corn in a saucepan of boiling water for 5 minutes. Drain and rinse under cold running water to cool; then drain again.
3 Preheat the broiler to medium. Thread the lamb, red bell peppers, zucchini, shallots, corn, and bay leaves onto four long skewers, dividing the ingredients equally between them.
4 Put the red wine, oil, mustard, garlic, and seasoning in a small bowl and whisk.
5 Arrange the kebabs on a broiler rack in a broiler pan and brush generously all over with the mustard mixture.

6 Broil for 10–15 minutes, turning occasionally, until the lambs and vegetables are cooked and tender. Brush the kebabs frequently with the mustard mixture to prevent them drying out.
7 Stir the chopped herbs and seasoning into the hot rice, then spoon the herbed rice onto a warmed serving dish. Place the cooked kebabs on top and serve with a mixed dark-green leaf salad.

Variations

- Use a mixture of wild rice and brown rice.
- Use unsweetened apple juice instead of red wine.
- Use button mushrooms instead of baby corn.
- Use pearl onions instead of shallots.

braised chicken *with* celery *and* mushrooms

Tender chicken breasts braised with celery and mushrooms, served with mashed potatoes or rice and cooked fresh vegetables, make a nutritious main meal. Chicken is a high-protein food, important for good brain function.

ingredients

- 1 tbsp olive oil
- 4 skinless, boneless chicken breasts
- 1 onion, sliced
- 6 celery stalks, sliced
- 2 parsnips, cut into large dice
- 8 ounces (225g) cremini mushrooms, sliced
- 8 ounces (225g) baby button mushrooms
- ⅓ cup/2 ounces (55g) whole green lentils
- 1¼ cups/½ pint (300ml) chicken stock (see recipe on page 20)
- ¾ cup/7 fl oz (200ml) dry or medium-dry white wine
- sea salt
- freshly ground black pepper
- 1 tbsp cornstarch (optional)
- 1 tbsp chopped fresh tarragon (optional)
- fresh herb sprigs, to garnish

serves *four*
preparation time *15 minutes*
cooking time *1 hour*

method

1 Preheat the oven to 350°F.
2 Heat the oil in a large flameproof, ovenproof casserole. Add the chicken and cook until sealed all over, turning occasionally. Remove the chicken from the casserole and set aside.
3 Add the onion and celery to the casserole and cook gently for 5 minutes, stirring occasionally.
4 Return the chicken to the casserole and add all the remaining ingredients, except the cornstarch, chopped tarragon, and herb garnish. Stir, then bring to a boil, stirring occasionally.
5 Cover and bake for about 1 hour, until the chicken, vegetables, and lentils are cooked and tender, stirring once or twice.
6 To thicken the sauce slightly, remove the chicken from the casserole with a slotted spoon. Place on a warmed plate, cover and keep hot. Blend the cornstarch with 2 tbsp water and stir into the casserole.

7 Bring slowly to a boil, stirring continuously, until the sauce thickens slightly; then simmer gently for 2 minutes, stirring. Stir in the chopped tarragon, if using.
8 Serve the hot chicken with the vegetable sauce spooned over.
9 Garnish with the herb sprigs and serve with fresh vegetables such as mashed potatoes and broccoli florets.

variations

- *Use small turkey breasts instead of chicken.*
- *Use 2 carrots instead of parsnips.*
- *Use 2 leeks instead of the onion.*
- *Use brown lentils instead of green.*

freezing instructions

Let cool completely, then transfer to a rigid, freezeproof container. Cover, seal, and label. Freeze for up to 3 months. Defrost for several hours, or overnight in the refrigerator. Reheat in the oven.

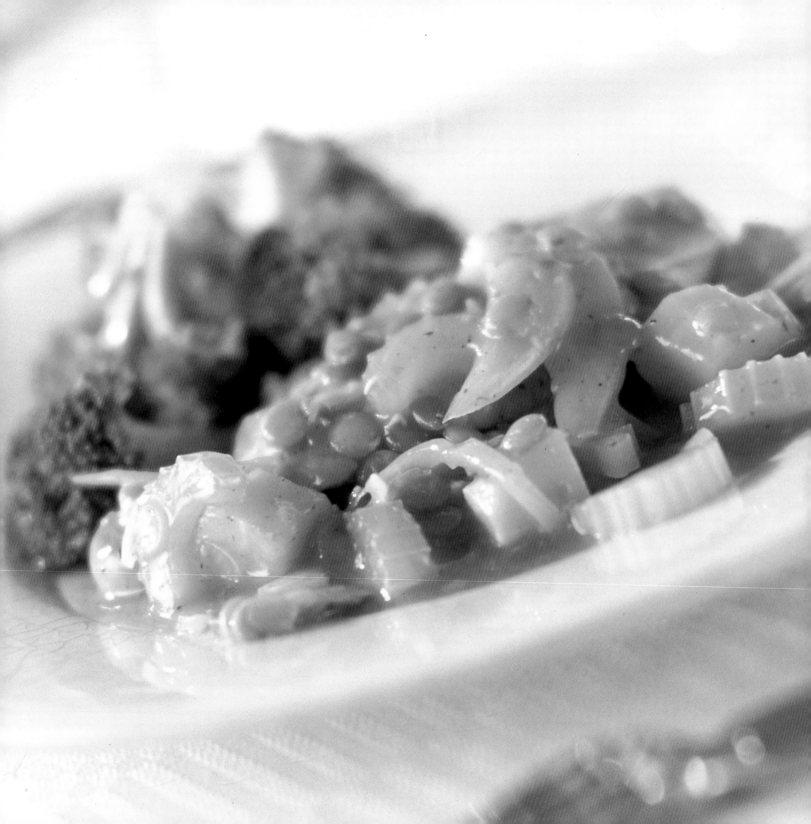

crunchy coleslaw *with* mustard dressing

Fresh raw vegetables, nuts, and dried fruits are tossed in a delicious mustard dressing to make this crunchy coleslaw. Nuts contain boron, which has been shown to improve mental alertness in deficient individuals.

ingredients

- 8 ounces (225g) green cabbage
- 8 ounces (225g) carrots
- 6 ounces (175g) small cauliflower florets
- ⅔ cup/4 ounces (115g) golden raisins
- ½ cup/3 ounces (85g) raisins
- ⅓ cup/2 ounces (55g) chopped, ready-to-eat dried peaches
- ¾ cup/3 ounces (85g) mixed nuts such as almonds, cashews, and pecans, chopped
- 6tbsp mayonnaise (see recipe on page 21)
- 6tbsp plain yogurt
- 1tbsp whole-grain mustard
- sea salt
- freshly ground black pepper
- fresh watercress sprigs, to garnish

serves *six*
preparation time *15 minutes, plus 1 hour chilling time*

method

1 Shred the cabbage and coarsely grate the carrots. Put them in a large serving bowl.
2 Halve the cauliflower florets and stir into the bowl with the mixed dried fruit and nuts.
3 Put the mayonnaise, yogurt, mustard, and seasoning in a small bowl and mix well.
4 Add the mayonnaise dressing to the cabbage mixture and mix well. Cover and refrigerate for at least 1 hour before serving.
5 Garnish with the watercress sprigs and serve with oven-baked potatoes topped with a little Cheddar or goat cheese.

variations

- *Use white or red cabbage instead of green cabbage.*
- *Use ready-to-eat dried apricots or pears instead of peaches.*
- *Add more dressing to taste.*

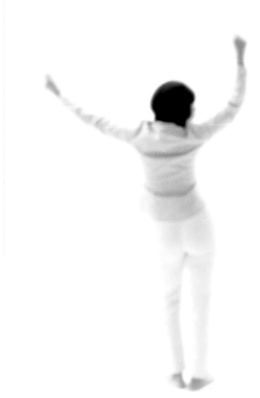

curried sweet potato *and* leek purée

This tasty purée of sweet potatoes and leeks, flavored with ground spices, is a tasty alternative to mashed potatoes. Sweet potatoes are a good source of beta carotene and vitamin C, both good brain foods.

ingredients

- 5 cups/1½ pounds (700g) diced sweet potatoes
- 2 cups/8 ounces (225g) washed and finely chopped leeks
- 1 tsp ground cumin
- 1 tsp ground coriander
- 1 tsp ground turmeric
- 1 clove garlic, crushed
- ½ cup/2 ounces (55g) finely grated Cheddar cheese
- 2 tbsp hot milk
- 1 tbsp chopped fresh cilantro
- sea salt
- freshly ground black pepper
- fresh cilantro sprigs, to garnish

serves *four*
preparation time *10 minutes*
cooking time *10–15 minutes*

method

1 Cook the potatoes in a saucepan of boiling water for 10–15 minutes, until cooked and tender. Drain thoroughly, then mash well until very smooth. Cover and keep hot.

2 Meanwhile, steam the leeks over a saucepan of boiling water for 10–15 minutes, until tender. Drain well, pressing out any excess water with the back of a spoon.

3 Add the leeks to the mashed potatoes with the ground spices, garlic, cheese, milk, cilantro, and seasoning, and mix well.

4 Garnish with the cilantro sprigs and serve with oven-roasted mixed vegetables or broiled lean meat or fish.

variations

- The ground spices can be omitted, or add 1–2 tsp curry powder instead.
- Use regular potatoes instead of sweet potatoes.
- Use chopped fresh parsley or basil instead of cilantro.

vegetable *dishes*

vegetable ragout *with* whole-wheat crust

 Serve this dough-topped vegetable ragout with new potatoes and green vegetables. Vegetables are a good source of vitamin C, which aids the absorption of iron—an essential nutrient for clear thinking.

ingredients

for the dough

- I cup/4 ounces (II5g) whole-wheat flour
- salt
- ¼ cup/2 ounces (55g) butter
- ¼ cup/I ounce (25g) finely grated, fresh Parmesan cheese,
- I tbsp chopped fresh chives
- I tbsp chopped parsley

for the ragout

- I onion, sliced
- I clove garlic, crushed
- I carrot, thinly sliced
- I zucchini, sliced
- 2 celery stalks, chopped
- I small green bell pepper, seeded and diced
- 4 ounces (II5g) mushrooms, sliced
- I I4-ounce (400g) can chopped tomatoes
- 4tbsp medium cider
- 2tsp dried mixed herbs
- ²⁄₃ cup/4 ounces (II5g) frozen peas
- salt and ground black pepper
- a little beaten egg, to glaze
- fresh herb sprigs, to garnish

serves *four*
preparation time *40 minutes*
cooking time *25–30 minutes*

method

I To make the dough, put the flour and a dash of salt in a bowl, then rub in the butter until the mixture resembles bread crumbs.
2 Stir in the Parmesan cheese and herbs; then add enough cold water to form a soft dough. Wrap and chill for 30 minutes.
3 Meanwhile, place all the remaining ingredients, except the seasoning, peas, beaten egg, and fresh herb garnish, in a large saucepan and stir. Cover and bring to a boil; then reduce the heat and simmer for 15 minutes, stirring occasionally. Uncover, increase the heat slightly, and cook for another 10 minutes, stirring occasionally.
4 Stir in the peas and season to taste with salt and pepper. Spoon the vegetables into an ovenproof pie dish.
5 Preheat the oven to 400°F.

6 Roll the dough out on a lightly floured surface to a shape a little larger than the pie dish.
7 Place the dough over the vegetable mixture in the pie plate, trim off excess and reserve the trimmings. Scallop or decorate the dough edges and make a hole in the center of the dough lid. Garnish the pie with dough trimmings and brush with a little beaten egg to glaze.
8 Bake for 25–30 minutes, until the dough is crisp and lightly browned.
9 Garnish with the herb sprigs and serve hot with fresh vegetables such as new potatoes and chopped spinach leaves or green beans.

variations

- *Use Cheddar cheese instead of Parmesan cheese.*
- *Use frozen fava beans instead of peas.*
- *Use I red or yellow bell pepper instead of green.*
- *Use white wine or vegetable stock instead of cider.*

vegetable *dishes*

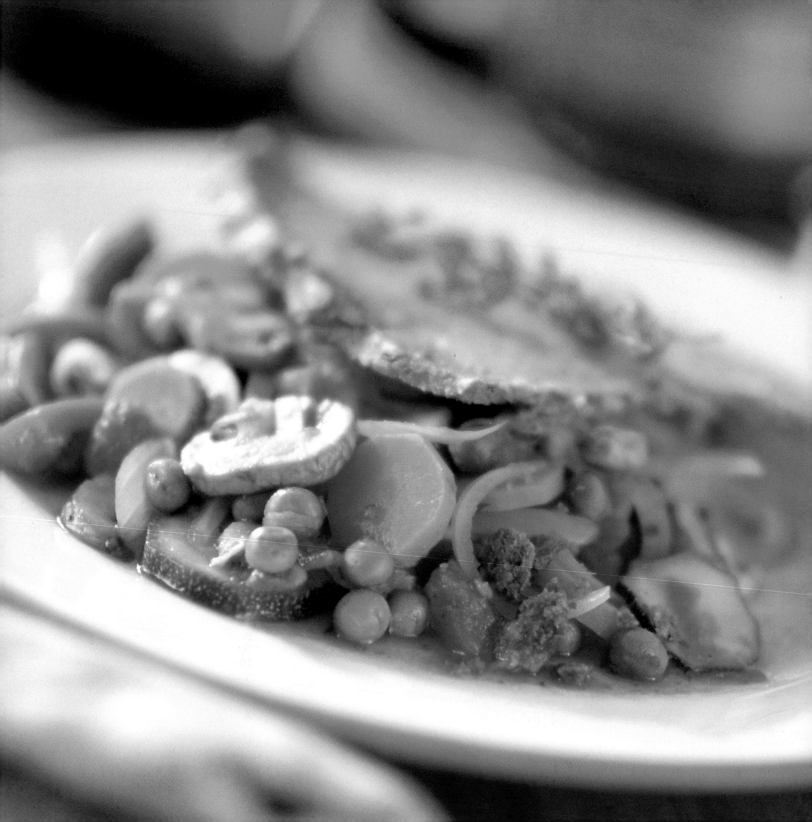

triple berry cobbler

 This delicious fruit dessert, served with homemade custard or yogurt, makes a popular family treat. Berries provide vitamin C, which is important for healthy brain function.

■ ingredients

- 1½ pounds (700g) mixed ripe raspberries, blackberries, and blueberries
- 2tbsp unsweetened apple juice
- ½ cup/4 ounces (115g) light brown sugar
- 1½ cups/6 ounces (175g) whole-wheat flour
- ⅔ cup/2 ounces (55g) uncooked oatmeal
- 2tsp baking powder
- 1tsp mixed ground spices
- ¼ cup/2 ounces (55g) butter, chopped
- 1 banana, peeled and mashed with a little lemon juice
- approx 4tbsp milk, plus extra for glazing

serves *four to six*
preparation time *20 minutes*
cooking time *15–20 minutes*

■ method

1 Preheat the oven to 425°F.
2 Put the berries and apple juice in a saucepan. Cover and cook gently for about 10 minutes, until softened. Remove the pan from the heat and stir in ¼ cup/ 2 ounces (55g) sugar. Transfer the berry mixture to an ovenproof dish.
3 Meanwhile, mix the flour, oatmeal, baking powder, and mixed spices in a bowl; then lightly rub in the chopped butter until the mixture resembles bread crumbs.
4 Stir in the remaining sugar; then stir in the mashed banana and enough milk to make a soft dough.
5 Turn the dough out onto a lightly floured surface and knead gently. Roll or pat out the dough and cut into 8 or 10 circles, using a 2-inch (5cm) fluted cutter.

6 Arrange the shapes around the edge of the ovenproof dish on top of the fruit, overlapping them slightly. Brush the dough with a little milk to glaze.
7 Bake for 15–20 minutes, until the dough is risen and golden brown.
8 Serve hot with homemade custard or yogurt.

variations

• Cut the dough into squares or triangles instead of circles.
• Use another fruit mixture such as apples, pears, and peaches instead of berries.
• Use ground cinnamon or ginger instead of mixed spice.

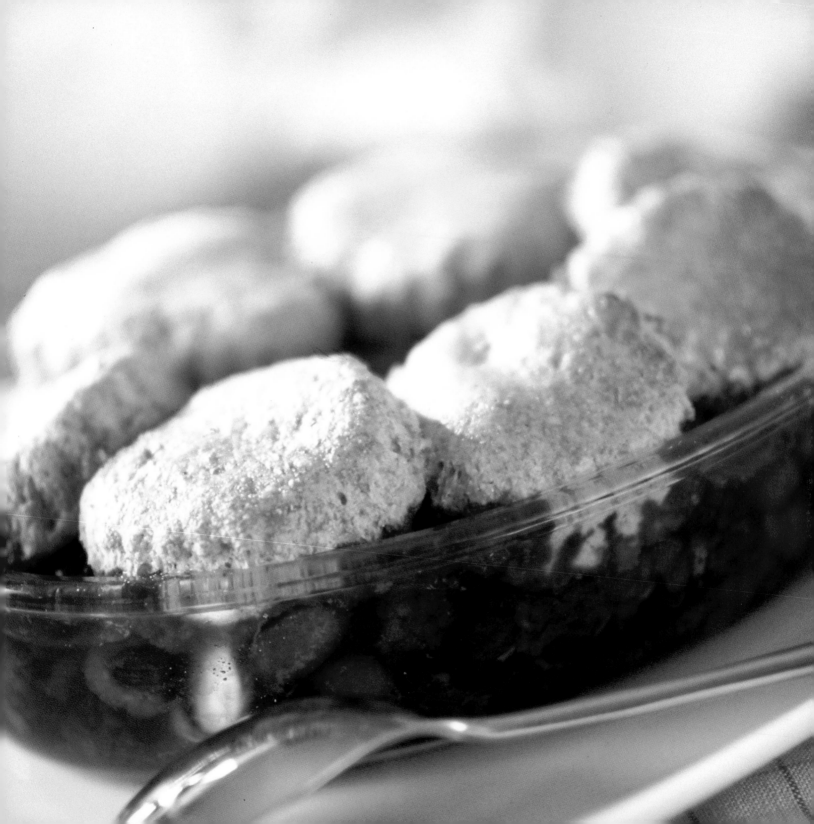

apple *and* apricot biscuit round

This fruity biscuit round is delicious spread with butter, honey, or jelly. Dried apricots contain minerals essential to a healthy brain.

■ ingredients

- 2 cups/8 ounces (225g) whole-wheat flour
- dash of salt
- 2tsp baking powder
- 1tsp ground cinnamon
- ¼ cup/2 ounces (55g) butter
- 2 tbsp/1 ounce (25g) light brown sugar
- ¾ cup/3 ounces (85g) finely chopped apricots
- 1 medium cooking apple, about 11 ounces (310g) in weight, peeled, cored, and coarsely grated
- approx 3–4tbsp milk, plus extra for glazing
- 1tbsp sugar

serves *eight*
preparation time *15 minutes*
cooking time *25–30 minutes*

■ method

1 Preheat the oven to 400°F.
2 Line a baking tray with nonstick baking paper.
3 Put the flour, salt, baking powder, and cinnamon in a bowl. Lightly rub in the chopped butter until the mixture resembles bread crumbs.
4 Stir in the sugar, apricots, apples, and enough milk to make a soft dough.
5 Turn the dough out onto a lightly floured surface. Knead gently and shape into a 7-inch (18cm) round. Place on the baking tray, brush with milk, and sprinkle with sugar. Mark into eight wedges.
6 Bake for 25–30 minutes, until risen and golden brown. Transfer to a wire rack to cool and break into wedges.
7 Serve warm or cold spread with butter, honey, or jelly.

variations

• *Use golden raisins or chopped ready-to-eat dried pineapple, pears, or peaches instead of apricots.*
• *Use ground mixed spices instead of cinnamon.*

blueberry brûlée

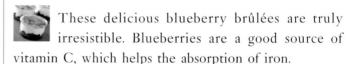

These delicious blueberry brûlées are truly irresistible. Blueberries are a good source of vitamin C, which helps the absorption of iron.

■ ingredients

- 12 ounces (350g) blueberries
- 1tbsp unsweetened apple juice
- 1tbsp honey
- ¾ cup/7 ounces (200g) plain yogurt
- ¾ cup/7 ounces (200g) crème fraîche
- ¼ cup/2 ounces (55g) sugar
- fresh mint sprigs, to decorate (optional)

serves *four to six*
preparation time *10 minutes, plus 3 hours' chilling time*
cooking time *15 minutes*

■ method

1 Put the blueberries in a saucepan with the apple juice and honey. Cover and cook gently for about 10 minutes, until the fruit is just softened. Remove the pan from the heat; uncover and set aside to cool completely.
2 When cool, spoon the blueberries into ramekins.
3 Fold the yogurt and crème fraîche together and spread evenly over the top of the blueberries, to cover completely. Chill for 3 hours.
4 Preheat the broiler to high. Sprinkle the sugar evenly over the yogurt mixture and place the dishes under the broiler for a few minutes, until the sugar melts and caramelizes. Cool and chill.
5 Decorate with fresh mint sprigs, if using, and serve with fresh fruit such as raspberries and peaches.

variations

• *Use blackberries or raspberries instead of blueberries.*
• *Use maple syrup instead of honey.*
• *Add 1tsp finely grated lemon or orange rind to the cooked fruit.*

desserts *and* bakes

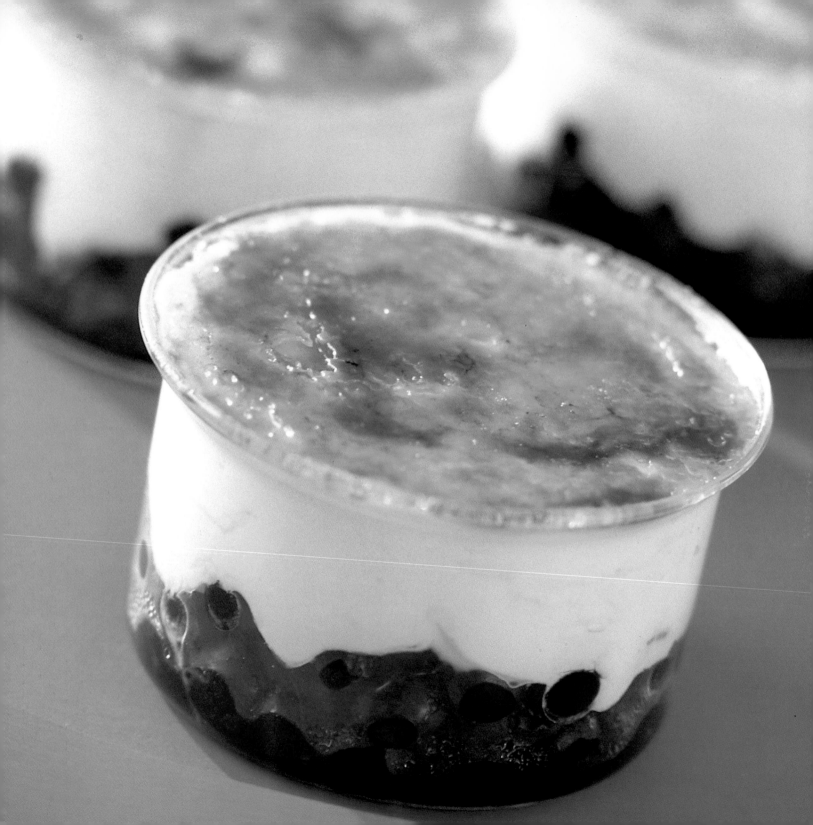

an interested party

THESE INSPIRING RECIPES *from the mental energy foods section contain all the nutrients you need to encourage clear thinking, such as* protein, *B* vitamins, vitamin *C, and the amino acid tyrosine which activates brain-stimulating chemicals. So eat up when you've got a tough assignment ahead.*

creamy carrot *and* celeriac soup

Kick off your meal with carrots for a good dose of B vitamins—vital nutrients for mental agility.

■ ingredients

- 2 tbsp/1 ounce (25g) butter
- 1 large onion, chopped
- 12 ounces (350g) carrots, sliced
- 2½/12 ounces (350g) diced celeriac
- 2½ cups/1 pint (600ml) vegetable stock (see recipe on page 20)
- sea salt and black pepper
- 1¼ cups/½ pint (300ml) milk
- 1–2tbsp chopped fresh cilantro
- fresh cilantro sprigs, to garnish

serves *four*
preparation time *15 minutes*
cooking time *40–45 minutes*

■ method

1 Melt the butter in a large saucepan. Add the onion, carrots and celeriac and cook gently for 5 minutes, stirring occasionally.
2 Add the stock and seasoning, and stir. Cover and bring to a boil; then reduce the heat and simmer for 30–40 minutes, until the vegetables are cooked and tender, stirring occasionally.
3 Remove the pan from the heat and set aside to cool slightly; then purée the soup in a blender or food processor until smooth.
4 Return the soup to the rinsed-out saucepan. Add the milk and chopped cilantro, if using, and reheat gently until piping hot, stirring occasionally.

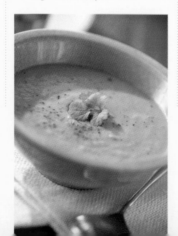

5 Ladle into warmed soup bowls to serve and garnish with fresh cilantro sprigs.
6 Serve with warm fresh whole-wheat bread rolls.

vegetable ragout *with* whole-wheat crust

The vegetables in this ragout provide vitamin C to help absorb the iron necessary to focus your thinking.

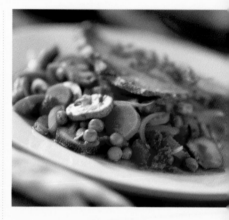

■ ingredients

- 1 onion, sliced
- 1 clove garlic, crushed
- 1 carrot, thinly sliced
- 1 zucchini, sliced
- 2 celery stalks, chopped
- 1 small green bell pepper, seeded and diced
- 4 ounces (115g) mushrooms, sliced
- 1 14-ounce (400g) can chopped tomatoes
- 4tbsp medium cider
- 2tsp dried mixed herbs
- salt
- freshly ground black pepper

- ²/₃ cup/4 ounces (115g) frozen peas
- a little beaten egg, to glaze
- fresh herb sprigs, to garnish

for the dough

- 1 cup/4 ounces (115g) whole-wheat flour
- salt
- ¼ cup/2 ounces (55g) butter
- ¼ cup/1 ounce (25g) finely grated, fresh Parmesan cheese,
- 1 tbsp chopped fresh chives
- 1 tbsp chopped parsley

serves *four*
preparation time *40 minutes*
cooking time *25–30 minutes*

method

1 To make the dough, put the flour and a dash of salt in a bowl, then rub in the butter until the mixture resembles bread crumbs.
2 Stir in the Parmesan cheese and herbs; then add enough cold water to form a soft dough. Wrap and chill for 30 minutes.
3 Meanwhile, place all the remaining ingredients, except the seasoning, peas, beaten egg, and fresh herb garnish, in a large saucepan and stir. Cover and bring to a boil; then reduce the heat and simmer for 15 minutes, stirring occasionally. Uncover, increase the heat slightly, and cook for another 10 minutes, stirring occasionally.
4 Stir in the peas and season to taste with salt and pepper. Spoon the vegetables into an ovenproof pie dish.
5 Preheat the oven to 400°F.
6 Roll the dough out on a lightly floured surface to a shape a little larger than the pie dish.
7 Place the dough over the vegetable mixture in the pie plate, trim off excess and reserve the trimmings. Scallop or decorate the dough edges and make a hole in the center of the dough lid. Garnish the pie with dough trimmings and brush with a little beaten egg to glaze.
8 Bake for 25–30 minutes, until the dough is crisp and lightly browned.
9 Garnish with the herb sprigs and serve hot with fresh vegetables such as new potatoes and chopped spinach leaves or green beans.

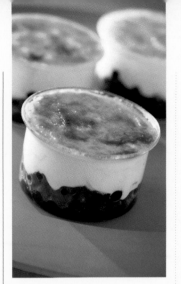

blueberry brûlée

As well as being high in vitamin C, blueberries are a nutritional bonus to aid iron absorption.

ingredients

- 12 ounces (350g) blueberries
- 1 tbsp unsweetened apple juice
- 1 tbsp honey
- ¾ cup/7 ounces (200g) plain yogurt
- ¾ cup/7 ounces (200g) crème fraîche
- ¼ cup/2 ounces (55g) sugar
- fresh mint sprigs, to decorate (optional)

serves *four to six*
preparation time *10 minutes, plus 3 hours' chilling time*
cooking time *15 minutes*

method

1 Put the blueberries in a saucepan with the apple juice and honey. Cover and cook gently for about 10 minutes, until the fruit is just softened. Remove the pan from the heat; uncover and set aside to cool completely.
2 When cool, spoon the blueberries into ramekins.
3 Fold the yogurt and crème fraîche together and spread evenly over the top of the blueberries, to cover completely. Chill for 3 hours.
4 Preheat the broiler to high. Sprinkle the sugar evenly over the yogurt mixture and place the dishes under the broiler for a few minutes, until the sugar melts and caramelizes. Cool and chill.
5 Decorate with fresh mint sprigs, if using, and serve with fresh fruit such as raspberries and peaches.

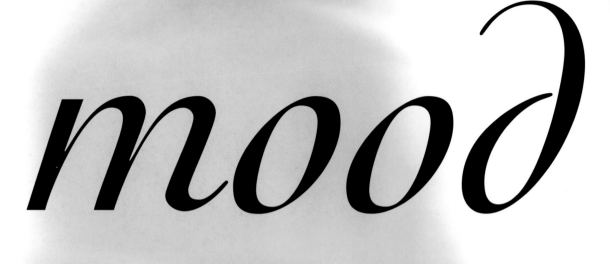

mood

In this Mood section we suggest nutritious recipes to balance your blood-sugar levels, which will help to reduce mood swings and feelings of lethargy. We encourage you to experiment and discover which foods suit your unique moods; whether you want to feel wide awake, inspired, or calm.

B-group vitamins are required to support normal brain functions. Vitamin B_3 (niacin), B_5 (pantothenic acid), B_6, and B_{12}, plus iron—another brilliant brain energizer—are all found in meats, poultry, eggs, fish, whole grains, and enriched cereals. Many of these foods also contain the amino acid tryptophan—known to relax the brain, reduce feelings of stress, and encourage deeper sleep. Magnesium and calcium are sometimes known as nature's tranquilizers, so if you want to remain calm and sleep well,

FOODS

try eating almonds, cashew nuts, cheese, yogurt, leafy green vegetables, legumes, and tofu, and before bed drink a glass of warm milk.

Vitamin C not only supports immune function within the body, it is also vital when the brain is tired or under stress. Mood swings, including some types of depression, may be signs of a deficiency of vitamins B and C. Citrus fruit, bell peppers, parsley, broccoli, lemons, and watercress are good sources of vitamin C. Seeds, nuts, and oily fish are rich in the essential fatty acids which are needed to make every cell and hormone within the body—and brain. Treats such as chocolate help to elevate mood as they contain a group of chemicals called endorphins that help you to feel good, but remember the magic words—balance in all things, even in your diet. Enjoy!

relaxing *foods*

IF YOU FEEL LIKE *a coiled spring at the end of the working day and need to wind down, then a dish featuring complex carbohydrates such as brown rice, pasta, noodles, couscous, or potato makes an ideal evening meal. A small bowl of muesli or any oat-based cereal, or a mashed banana with yogurt, about an hour before bedtime, can encourage sounder sleep. By eating complex carbohydrates you can increase levels of serotonin, the brain chemical that is known for its calming and soothing properties. Feelings of serenity, security, and tranquility are all associated with adequate levels of serotonin.*

green salad *with* avocado dressing

Serve this refreshing salad with whole-wheat bread as an appetizer or snack. Dark green salad leaves are rich in many nutrients including iron, B vitamins, vitamin C, calcium, and magnesium, all of which are needed for brain function.

ingredients

- 5 ounces (140g) mixed dark-green salad leaves such as baby spinach, lollo rosso (coral lettuce), red (ruby) chard, and rocket
- ½ cup/2 ounces (55g) watercress
- 1 green bell pepper, seeded and sliced
- half an English cucumber, thinly sliced
- 1 bunch green onions, chopped
- ½–⅓ cup/2–3 ounces (55–85g) roughly chopped walnuts

for the dressing

- 1 large avocado
- finely grated rind and juice of 1 lemon
- 6tbsp plain yogurt
- 1tsp Dijon mustard
- sea salt
- freshly ground black pepper

serves *four to six*
preparation time *15 minutes*

method

1 Put the salad leaves in a large bowl. Add the watercress, green pepper, cucumber, and green onions, and toss together. Divide the salad among four to six serving plates or bowls.
2 To make the dressing, peel, pit, and chop the avocado and place in a food processor with the lemon rind and juice. Blend until smooth. Add the yogurt, mustard, and seasoning, and blend.
3 Spoon some dressing over each salad. Sprinkle with the walnuts and serve with crusty whole-wheat bread.

variation

• *Use the finely grated rind and juice of 1 lime instead of the lemon.*

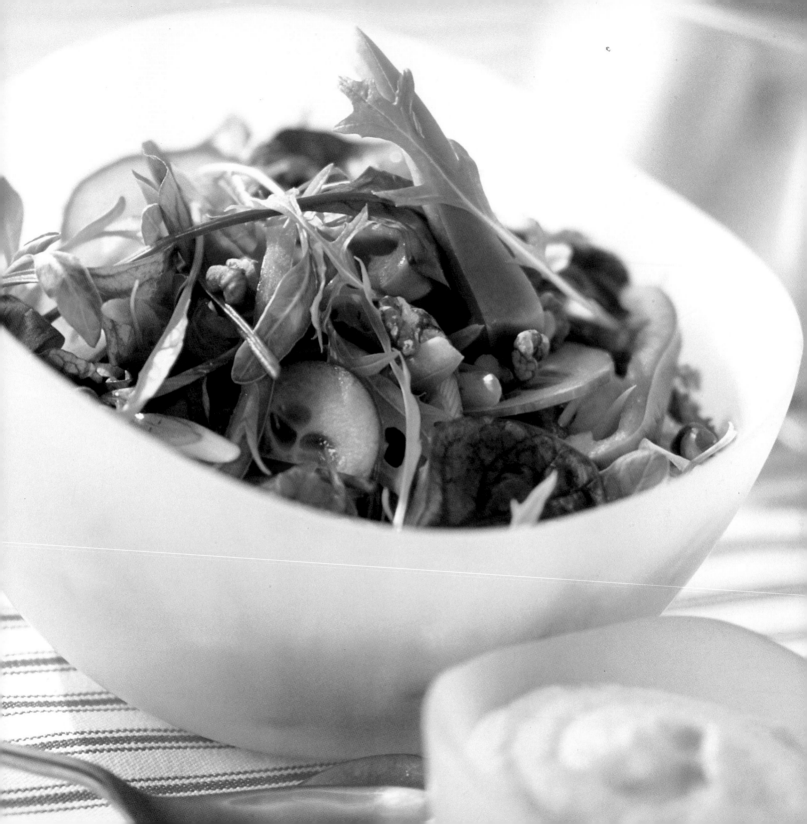

summer lettuce soup

This refreshing summer soup makes an ideal appetizer or light lunch. Lettuce contains beta carotene, potassium, vitamin C, and some calcium. It is often used by herbalists as a calming food.

ingredients

- 1tbsp olive oil
- 1 onion, chopped
- 1½ cups/8 ounces (225g) diced potatoes
- 4 cups/8 ounces (225g) shredded round (butterhead) lettuce,
- 1¼ cups/½ pint (300ml) chicken stock (see recipe on page 20)
- 1¼ cups/½ pint (300ml) milk
- sea salt
- freshly ground black pepper
- 2tbsp chopped fresh parsley
- 2tbsp light (pouring) cream, to garnish (optional)

serves *four*
preparation time *10 minutes*
cooking time *25–30 minutes*

method

1 Heat the oil in a large saucepan. Add the onion and potatoes, and cook gently for 5 minutes, stirring occasionally, until soft.
2 Add the lettuce and cook gently for 2 minutes; then add the stock, milk, seasoning, and stir.
3 Cover and bring to a boil; then reduce the heat and simmer for 10 minutes, stirring occasionally, until the vegetables are tender.
4 Remove the pan from the heat and let cool slightly; then blend the soup in a blender or food processor until smooth.
5 Return the soup to the rinsed-out saucepan and stir in the chopped parsley; then reheat gently until piping hot, stirring occasionally.
6 Ladle into warmed soup bowls to serve and garnish each serving with a swirl of cream, if liked.
7 Serve with whole-wheat rolls.

variations

- *Use spinach instead of lettuce.*
- *Use sweet potatoes instead of regular potatoes.*
- *Use 1 leek instead of the onion.*

freezing instructions

Let cool completely, then transfer to a rigid, freezeproof container. Cover, seal, and label. Freeze for up to 3 months. Defrost for several hours, or overnight in the refrigerator. Reheat gently in a saucepan until piping hot.

poached eggs *with* tuna salad

Poached eggs served with tuna salad makes an appetizing snack or first course. Tuna provides iron and magnesium, which are vital for a healthy nervous system. Yogurt, like other forms of milk, contains tryptophan, which the brain converts into the soothing chemical serotonin.

■ ingredients

- 1 6-ounce (185g) can tuna in water, drained and mashed
- 4tbsp mayonnaise (see recipe on page 21)
- 2tbsp plain yogurt
- 2 green onions, finely chopped
- 1tsp finely grated lemon rind
- sea salt
- freshly ground black pepper
- 4 medium eggs
- shredded round (butterhead) lettuce leaves and watercress, to garnish

serves *four*
preparation time *10 minutes*
cooking time *4–6 minutes*

■ method

1 Put the tuna, mayonnaise, yogurt, green onions, lemon rind, and seasoning in a bowl and mix thoroughly. Cover and chill while poaching the eggs.

2 Fill a skillet or saucepan with water to a depth of about 3 inches (7.5cm). Bring to a boil; then swirl the water with a spoon and slip the eggs into the water, one by one. Cook gently for a few minutes until lightly set, or longer if you prefer firmer eggs.

3 Carefully remove the eggs from the pan using a slotted spoon and place each one on a serving plate. Spoon some tuna salad alongside and garnish each serving with a little shredded lettuce and watercress.

4 Serve with crispbread or slices of whole-wheat toast.

variations

- *Boil the eggs instead of poaching.*
- *Spread the tuna salad over whole-wheat toast and top with a poached egg.*
- *Add 1 small clove garlic, crushed, to the tuna salad.*
- *Use canned red or pink salmon instead of tuna.*

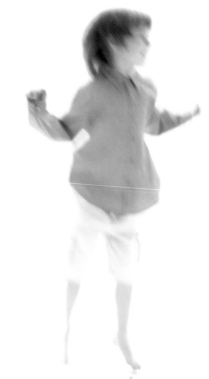

soups and appetizers

salmon, pepper, *and* mushroom whole-wheat pizza

Pizzas are always a popular family meal, and the addition of salmon provides extra B vitamins, which help to maintain a healthy nervous system. Fresh vegetables are rich in vitamin C, so you can replenish your stock with the pepper and tomato on this delicious pizza.

■ ingredients

- 1 tbsp olive oil
- 4 shallots (French shallots), sliced
- 1 red bell pepper, seeded and sliced
- 8 ounces (225g) mushrooms, sliced
- 1 clove garlic, crushed
- 4 tbsp crushed tomatoes
- 4 sun-dried tomatoes in oil, drained and finely chopped
- 1–2 tbsp chopped fresh mixed herbs
- sea salt
- freshly ground black pepper
- 1 7-ounce (213g) can salmon in water, drained and flaked
- 2 plum (Roma) tomatoes, sliced
- 1 cup/4 ounces (115g) grated Cheddar cheese
- fresh herb sprigs, to garnish

for the pizza dough

- 1½ cups/6 ounces (175g) whole-wheat flour
- ½ cup/2 ounces (55g) uncooked oatmeal
- dash of salt
- 2 tsp baking powder
- ¼ cup/2 ounces (55g) butter
- scant ½ cup/13 fluid ounces (100ml) milk

serves *four to six*
preparation time *25 minutes*
cooking time *25–30 minutes*

■ method

1 Preheat the oven to 425°F.
2 Line a baking tray with nonstick baking paper.
3 Heat the oil in a saucepan. Add the shallots, pepper, mushrooms, and garlic. Cook gently for 10 minutes, stirring occasionally, until soft.
4 Meanwhile, make the pizza dough. Put the flour, oatmeal, salt, and baking powder in a bowl and lightly rub in the butter until the mixture resembles bread crumbs. Add enough milk to make a soft but not sticky dough.
5 Roll the dough out on a lightly floured surface to a circle roughly 10 inches (25cm) in diameter. Place the dough on the baking tray and make the edges slightly thicker than the center.
6 Mix the crushed tomatoes, sun-dried tomatoes, chopped herbs, and seasoning together and spread over the pizza base.
7 Spoon the cooked vegetables over the base, scatter over the salmon, and top with the tomato slices. Sprinkle the cheese evenly over the top.
8 Bake for 25–30 minutes, until cooked and golden brown.
9 Garnish with the herb sprigs and serve hot or cold with crusty whole-wheat bread and a pepper and tomato salad.

variations

- *Use canned tuna instead of salmon.*
- *Use zucchini or eggplants instead of mushrooms.*

freezing instructions

Let cool completely; then wrap in foil, seal, and label. Freeze for up to 3 months. Defrost for several hours, or overnight in the refrigerator. Reheat in a moderate oven.

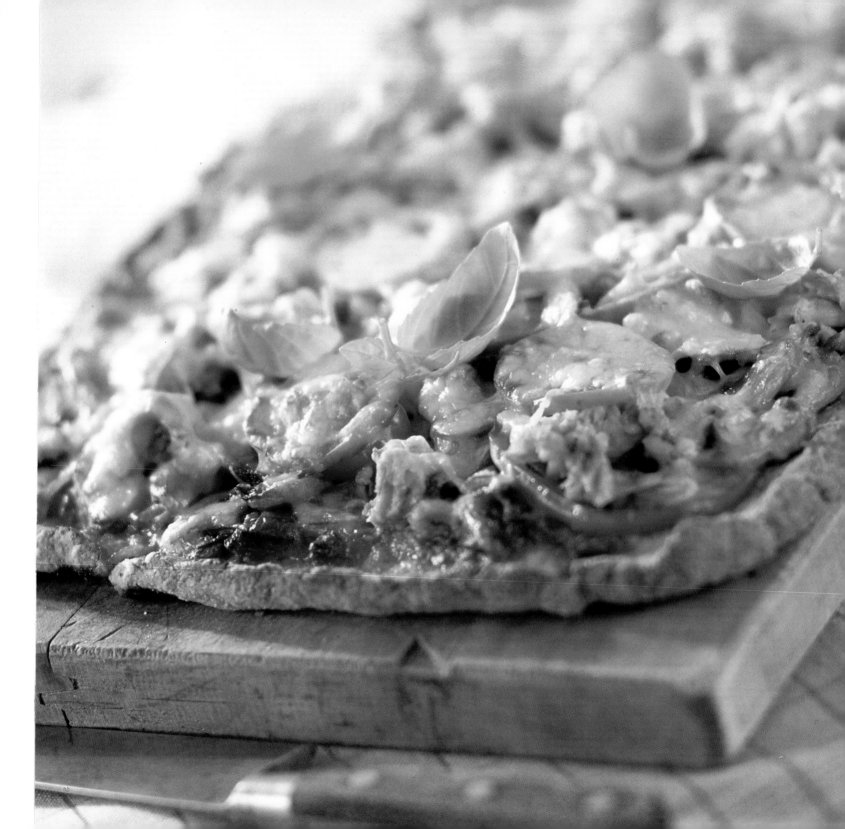

barbecued chicken *with* shallots

This chicken dish, served with a hot and spicy relish, can be cooked on a barbecue or in the oven. Chicken is a good source of protein and B vitamins, which are essential for healthy brain function.

■ ingredients

- 3tbsp olive oil
- 1tbsp cajun seasoning
- 6 skinless chicken legs or breast portions
- 1 pound (450g) shallots (French shallots), halved
- fresh herb sprigs, to garnish

for the relish

- 1 14-ounce (400g) can tomatoes, chopped
- 1 onion, finely chopped
- 1 small fresh red chili, seeded and finely chopped
- 1 clove garlic, crushed
- 1tbsp light brown sugar
- 1tbsp Worcestershire sauce
- 1tbsp red wine vinegar
- 1tbsp tomato paste
- ½tsp English mustard
- sea salt
- freshly ground black pepper

serves *six*
preparation time *10 minutes*
cooking time *45 minutes*

■ method

1 Preheat the oven to 400°F.

2 Mix the oil and cajun seasoning in a bowl. Place the chicken portions and shallots in a roasting pan and brush with the oil.

3 Bake for about 45 minutes, until the chicken is cooked through and tender.

4 Meanwhile, put all the relish ingredients in a saucepan and stir. Bring to a boil; then simmer, uncovered, for 15–20 minutes, until the sauce is cooked and thickened, stirring occasionally.

5 Put the cooked chicken and shallots onto warmed serving plates. Spoon some relish alongside and garnish with the herb sprigs.

6 Serve with cooked fresh vegetables such as baby (Dutch) carrots, zucchini, and oven-baked potatoes.

variations

• *Cook the chicken on hot barbecue coals instead of in the oven.*

• *Use ½–1 tsp hot chili powder instead of the fresh chili.*

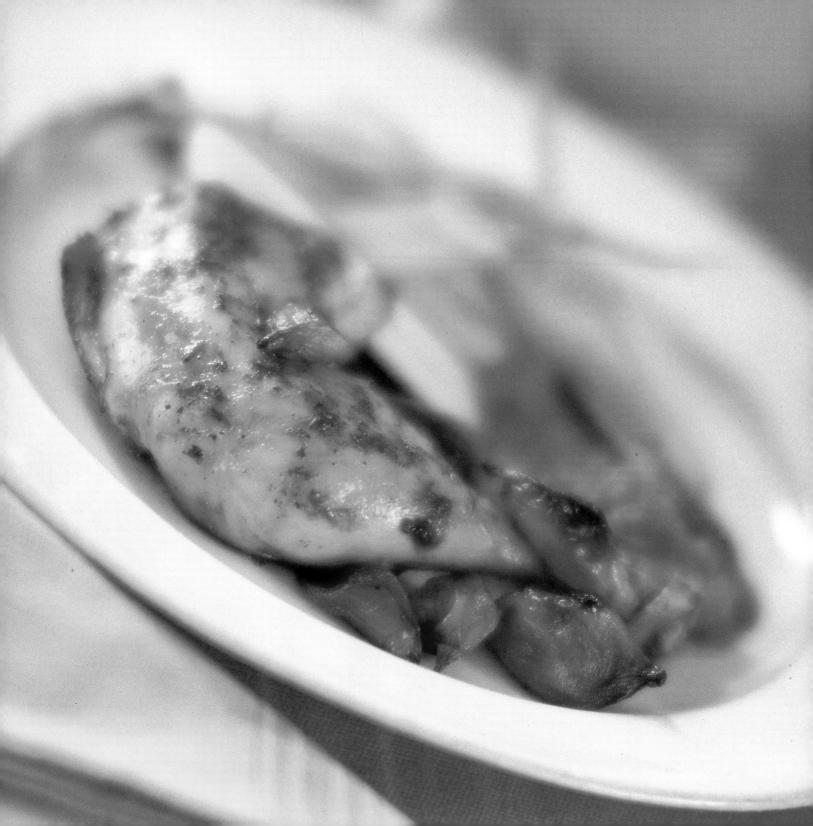

root vegetable rösti

The swiss word *rösti* means "crisp and golden." Try this rösti of root vegetables for an appetizing side dish or light meal. High-carbohydrate root vegetables can help boost serotonin, the stress-busting, tranquilizing hormone. Fresh chives contain vitamin C and a little iron.

ingredients

- 8 ounces (225g) medium-size potatoes
- 2 medium carrots
- 2 small parsnips
- 2tbsp chopped fresh chives
- sea salt
- freshly ground black pepper
- 2tbsp olive oil
- 1 small onion, finely chopped
- fresh chives, to garnish

serves *four*
preparation time *15 minutes*
cooking time *15–20 minutes*

method

1 Peel the potatoes, carrots, and parsnips and cook them in a saucepan of lightly salted, boiling water for 6 minutes. Drain well and set aside to cool.

2 When cool enough to handle, grate the parboiled vegetables into a bowl and stir in the chopped chives and seasoning.

3 Heat the oil in a 10-inch (25cm) nonstick skillet. Add the onion and cook for about 5 minutes, until softened, stirring occasionally.

4 Add the vegetable mixture and stir; then shape into a cake the size of the skillet, pressing down gently. Fry over a medium heat until golden brown underneath.

5 Carefully turn the cake over using a wide spatula, or turn it out onto a plate and slide it back into the skillet. Cook until the other side is browned and crisp.

6 Cut into wedges and garnish with the chives.

7 Serve with cooked fresh vegetables such as green beans and baby spinach leaves.

variations

- *Use sweet potatoes instead of regular potatoes.*
- *Use rutabaga instead of carrots.*
- *Use chopped fresh parsley or mixed herbs instead of chives.*

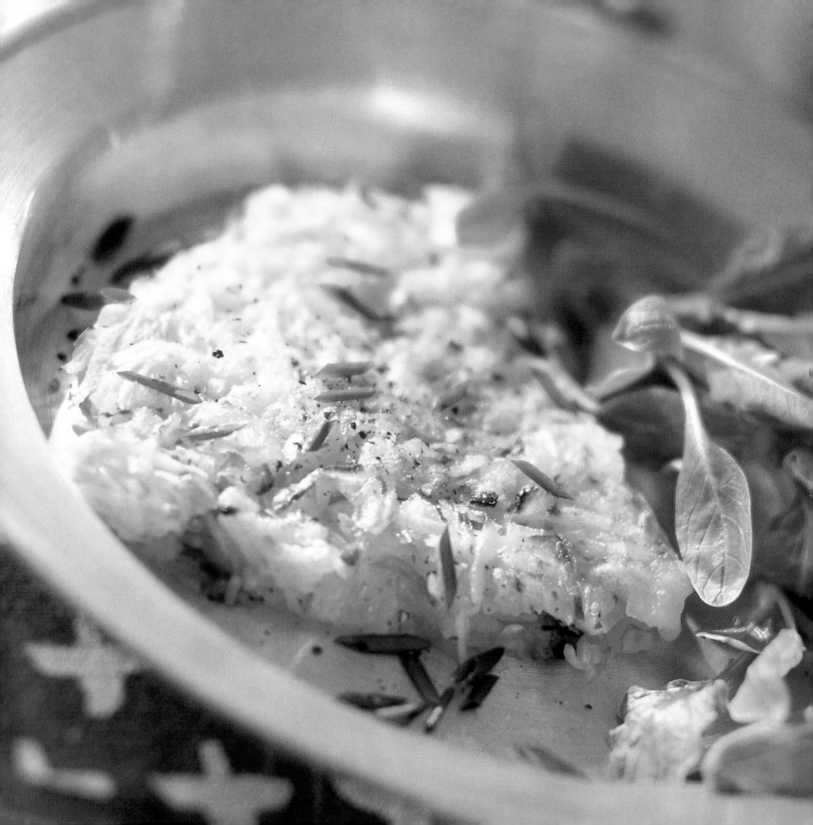

tomato *and* basil penne

Freshly cooked pasta served with a delicious tomato sauce makes a quick, delicious meal. The complex carbohydrates found in pasta may increase levels of serotonin, a chemical known for its calming properties. Serotonin can also help ease anxiety and increase the ability to wind down.

ingredients

- 1 tbsp olive oil
- 6 shallots (French shallots), finely chopped
- 2 cloves garlic, finely chopped
- 2 celery stalks, finely chopped
- 3 cups/1 pound 9 ounces (700g) peeled, seeded, and chopped tomatoes
- 4 sun-dried tomatoes, soaked, drained and finely chopped
- 2 tbsp medium-dry sherry
- 1 tbsp tomato paste
- ½ tsp light brown sugar
- sea salt
- freshly ground black pepper
- 12 ounces (350g) penne pasta
- 2–3 tbsp chopped fresh basil
- freshly grated Parmesan cheese, to serve
- fresh basil sprigs, to garnish

serves *four*
preparation time *15 minutes*
cooking time *30–35 minutes*

method

1 Heat the oil in a saucepan. Add the shallots, garlic, and celery, and cook gently for 5 minutes, stirring occasionally, until soft.

2 Add the tomatoes, sun-dried tomatoes, sherry, tomato paste, sugar, and seasoning, and mix well. Cover and bring to a boil; then reduce the heat and simmer for 15 minutes, stirring occasionally.

3 Uncover, increase the heat slightly, and cook for another 10–15 minutes, until the mixture is cooked and thickened.

4 Meanwhile, cook the pasta in a large saucepan of lightly salted, boiling water, for 10–12 minutes, until just cooked or *al dente*.

5 Drain the pasta well; then toss the pasta, tomato sauce, and chopped basil together.

6 Serve hot, sprinkled with a little Parmesan cheese and garnished with the basil sprigs.

7 Serve with a mixed dark-green leaf side salad.

variations

- *Use leeks instead of shallots.*
- *Use carrots instead of celery.*
- *Use chopped fresh mixed herbs instead of basil.*

vegetable *dishes*

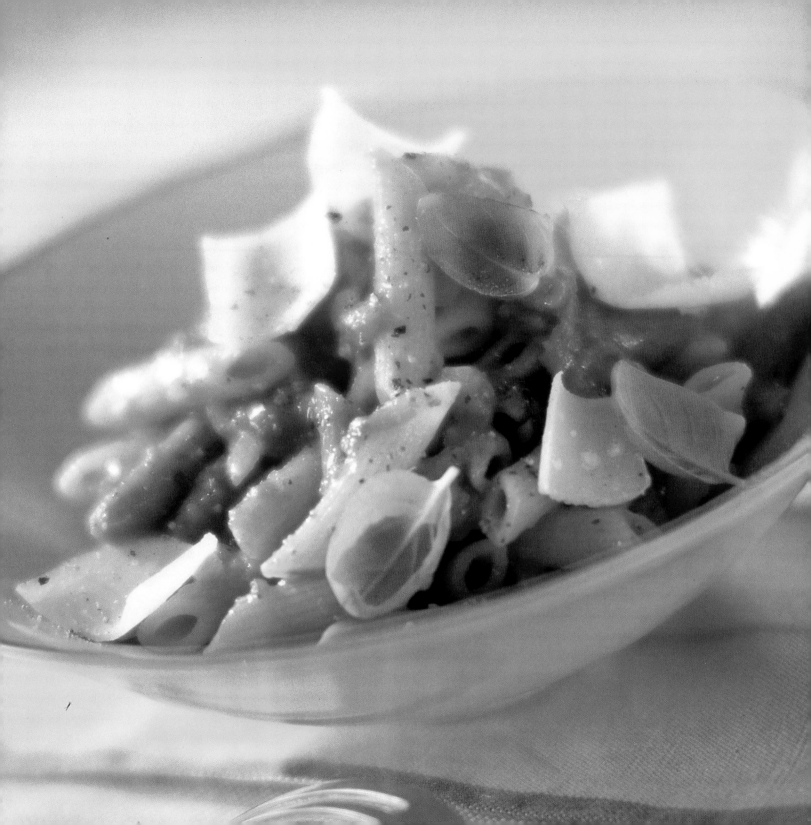

raspberry *and* apple oatmeal crumble

This fruit crumble is good served with homemade custard or a little vanilla yogurt. Fresh fruits such as raspberries and apples are a good source of vitamin C, a vital vitamin for anyone suffering from stress.

ingredients

- 1 cup/4 ounces (115g) whole-wheat flour
- ¾ cup/3 ounces (85g) uncooked oatmeal
- ⅓ cup/3 ounces (85g) butter, chopped
- ½ cup/4 ounces (115g) light brown sugar
- 8 ounces (225g) fresh raspberries
- 8 ounces (225g) eating apples peeled, cored, and thinly sliced
- 1 tsp ground cinnamon

serves *four*
preparation time *15 minutes*
cooking time *45 minutes*

method

1 Preheat the oven to 350°F.
2 Mix the flour and oatmeal in a bowl; then rub in the butter; until the mixture resembles bread crumbs. Stir in ⅓ cup/3 ounces (85g) of the brown sugar.
3 Put the raspberries and apples in an ovenproof dish. Mix the remaining sugar and cinnamon, and sprinkle over the fruit.
4 Spoon the oatmeal mixture evenly over the fruit.
5 Bake in the preheated oven for about 45 minutes, until the fruit is cooked and the topping is golden brown.
6 Serve hot or cold with homemade custard or vanilla yogurt.

variations

- *Use other tasty combinations of fresh fruits, such as peaches and raspberries, apples and pears, or apricots and pineapple.*
- *Use ground mixed spice or ginger instead of cinnamon.*

freezing instructions

Let cool completely, then transfer to a rigid, freezeproof container. Cover, seal, and label. Freeze for up to 3 months. Defrost for several hours, or overnight in the refrigerator. Reheat in the oven.

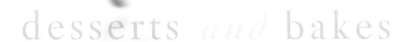

desserts *and* bakes

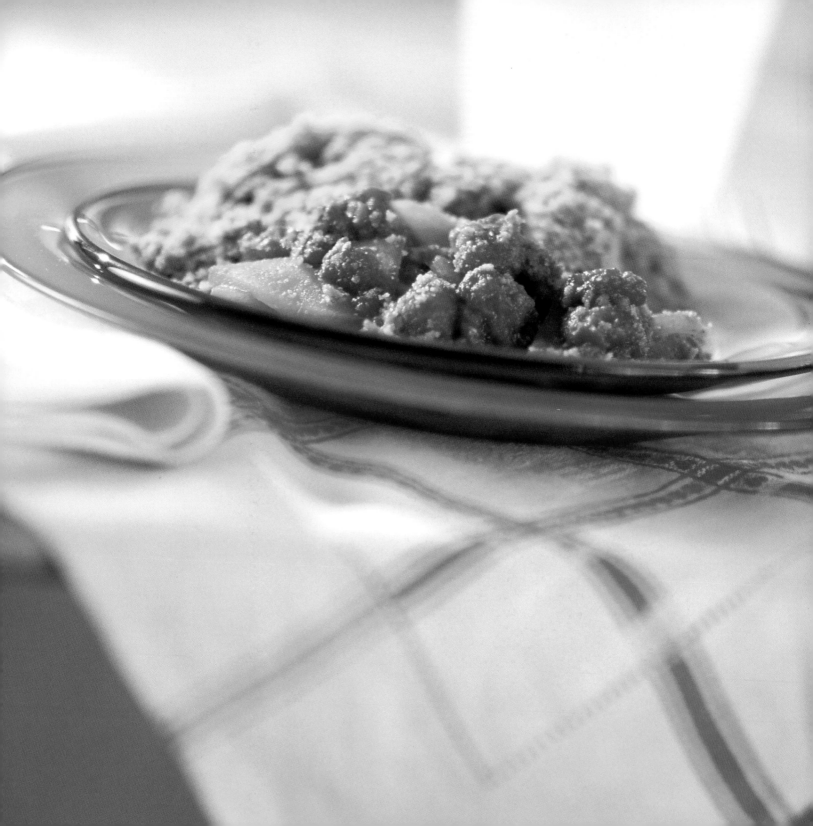

date *and* raisin snack bars

 These chewy, fruity snack bars are ideal for a packed lunch. Oats help the body produce the calming hormone serotonin. Dried fruit contains iron and magnesium.

■ ingredients

- ½ cup/4 ounces (115g) butter
- ⅓ cup/3 ounces (85g) light brown sugar
- 3tbsp maple syrup
- ¾ cup/3 ounces (85g) rolled oats
- ¾ cup/3 ounces (85g) sugar-free Swiss-style muesli
- ⅓ cup/2 ounces (55g) finely chopped dried dates
- ⅓ cup/2 ounces (55g) raisins

makes *8–10 bars*
preparation time *15 minutes*
cooking time *20–30 minutes*

■ method

1 Preheat the oven to 350°F.
2 Lightly grease a shallow 7-inch (18cm) square cake pan.
3 Put the butter, sugar, and syrup in a saucepan and heat gently until melted. Remove from the heat.
4 Stir in the oats, muesli, dates, and raisins, and mix well.
5 Transfer the mixture to the prepared pan, pressing it down well to level the surface.
6 Bake for 20–30 minutes, until pale golden brown. Mark into fingers or squares while still warm, then let cool completely in the pan.
7 When cool, break into fingers or squares.

variations

• *Use honey instead of maple syrup.*
• *Use ready-to-eat dried apricots and apples instead of dates and raisins.*
• *Add 1 tsp ground mixed spices, ginger, or cinnamon to the mixture before baking.*

fruit salad *with* ginger

Quick and easy to make, this fresh fruit salad provides a delicious and refreshing end to any meal. Ginger is known to be calming to a stressed or overworked digestive system.

■ ingredients

- 1 small melon
- 6 kiwi fruit
- 2–3 pieces/1 ounce (25g) preserved stem ginger in syrup, drained
- ¾ cup/7 fluid ounces (200ml) unsweetened apple juice
- scant ½ cup/3 fluid ounces (100ml) unsweetened white grape juice
- 2tbsp ginger wine
- fresh mint sprigs, to garnish

serves *four*
preparation time *15 minutes, plus 1 hour standing time*

■ method

1 Halve the melon; discard the seeds. Peel the melon and dice the flesh. Place it in a bowl.
2 Peel and slice the kiwi fruit and finely chop the stem ginger. Add to the bowl and stir.
3 Mix the fruit juices and ginger wine. Pour over the fruit and stir; then cover and leave to stand at room temperature for 1 hour before serving to let the flavors blend.
4 Garnish with the mint sprigs and serve with a little plain yogurt.

variations

• *Use 1 small fresh pineapple instead of the melon.*
• *Use a mixture of unsweetened orange and pineapple juices instead of the apple and grape juices.*
• *Use brandy or sherry instead of ginger wine.*

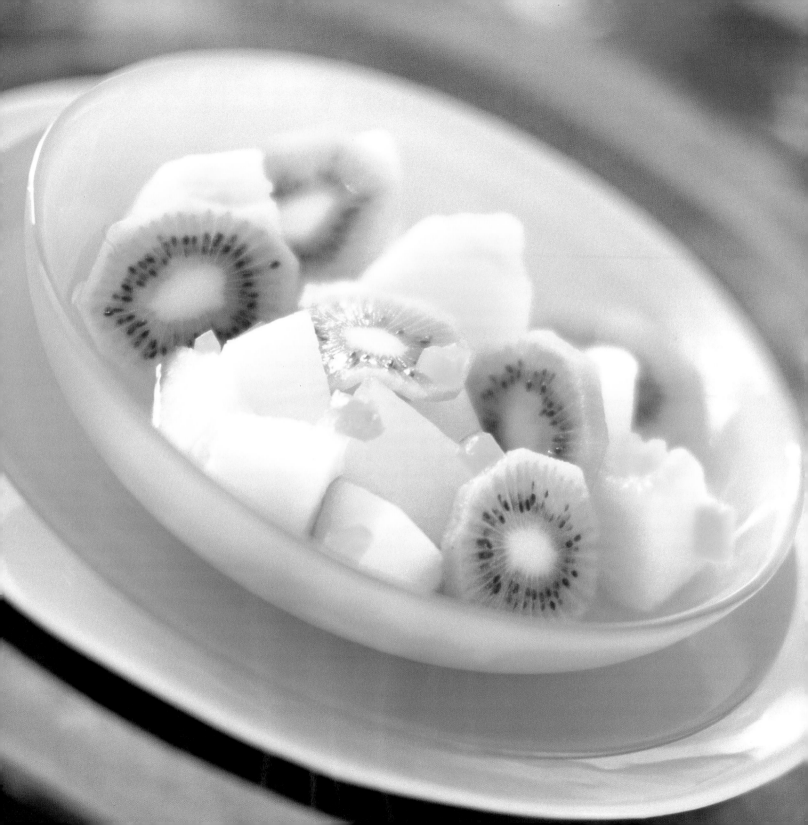

easy like sunday morning

SIT BACK AND RELAX *with this selection of meals from the relaxing foods section. These recipes are rich in nutrients that increase levels* of the stress-busting and tranquilizing hormones serotonin and tryptophan. So settle down to a nutritious feast that will calm and soothe away the strain of the day.

green salad *with* avocado dressing

A fabulous mind soother, this salad contains a whole host of vitamins and minerals to help improve your mental state.

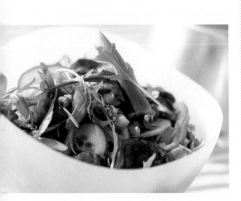

ingredients

- 5 ounces (140g) mixed dark-green salad leaves such as baby spinach, lollo rosso (coral lettuce), red (ruby) chard, and rocket
- ½ cup/2 ounces (55g) watercress
- 1 green bell pepper, seeded and sliced
- half an English cucumber, thinly sliced
- 1 bunch green onions, chopped
- ½–⅓ cup/2–3 ounces (55–85g) roughly chopped walnuts

for the dressing

- 1 large avocado
- finely grated rind and juice of 1 lemon
- 6tbsp plain yogurt
- 1tsp Dijon mustard
- sea salt
- freshly ground black pepper

serves *four to six*
preparation time *15 minutes*

method

1 Put the salad leaves in a large bowl. Add the watercress, green pepper, cucumber, and green onions, and toss together. Divide the salad among four to six serving plates or bowls.
2 To make the dressing, peel, pit, and chop the avocado and place in a food processor with the lemon rind and juice. Blend until smooth. Add the yogurt, mustard, and seasoning, and blend.
3 Spoon some dressing over each salad. Sprinkle with the walnuts and serve with crusty whole-wheat bread.

salmon, pepper, *and* mushroom whole-wheat pizza

The B vitamins in this pizza make this main course an excellent de-stresser.

ingredients

- 1tbsp olive oil
- 4 shallots (French shallots), sliced
- 1 red bell pepper, seeded and sliced
- 8 ounces (225g) mushrooms, sliced
- 1 clove garlic, crushed
- 4tbsp crushed tomatoes
- 4 sun-dried tomatoes in oil, drained and finely chopped
- 1–2tbsp chopped fresh mixed herbs
- sea salt

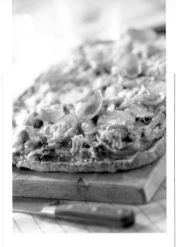

- freshly ground black pepper
- 1 7-ounce (213g) can salmon in water, drained and flaked
- 2 plum (Roma) tomatoes, sliced
- 1 cup/4 ounces (115g) grated Cheddar cheese
- fresh herb sprigs, to garnish

for the pizza dough

- 1½ cups/6 ounces (175g) whole-wheat flour
- ½ cup/2 ounces (55g) uncooked oatmeal
- dash of salt
- 2tsp baking powder
- ¼ cup/2 ounces (55g) butter
- scant ½ cup/13 fluid ounces (100ml) milk

serves *four to six*
preparation time *25 minutes*
cooking time *25–30 minutes*

method

1 Preheat the oven to 425°F.
2 Line a baking tray with nonstick baking paper.
3 Heat the oil in a saucepan. Add the shallots, pepper, mushrooms, and garlic. Cook gently for

10 minutes, stirring occasionally, until soft.
4 Meanwhile, make the pizza dough. Put the flour, oatmeal, salt, and baking powder in a bowl and lightly rub in the butter until the mixture resembles bread crumbs. Add enough milk to make a soft but not sticky dough.
5 Roll the dough out on a lightly floured surface to a circle roughly 10 inches (25cm) in diameter. Place the dough on the baking tray and make the edges slightly thicker than the center.
6 Mix the crushed tomatoes, sun-dried tomatoes, chopped herbs, and seasoning together and spread over the pizza base.
7 Spoon the cooked vegetables over the base, scatter over the salmon, and top with the tomato slices. Sprinkle the cheese evenly over the top.
8 Bake for 25–30 minutes, until cooked and golden brown.
9 Garnish with the herb sprigs and serve hot or cold with crusty whole-wheat bread and a pepper and tomato salad.

raspberry *and* apple oatmeal crumble

Boost your vitamin C stores with the raspberries and apples in this nutritious dessert.

ingredients

- 1 cup/4 ounces (115g) whole-wheat flour
- ¾ cup/3 ounces (85g) uncooked oatmeal
- ⅓ cup/3 ounces (85g) butter, chopped
- ½ cup/4 ounces (115g) light brown sugar
- 8 ounces (225g) fresh raspberries
- 8 ounces (225g) eating apples peeled, cored, and thinly sliced
- 1tsp ground cinnamon

serves *four*
preparation time *15 minutes*
cooking time *45 minutes*

method

1 Preheat the oven to 350°F.
2 Mix the flour and oatmeal in a bowl; then rub in the butter; until the mixture resembles bread crumbs. Stir in ⅓ cup/3 ounces (85g) of the brown sugar.
3 Put the raspberries and apples in an ovenproof dish. Mix the remaining sugar and cinnamon, and sprinkle over the fruit.
4 Spoon the oatmeal mixture evenly over the fruit.
5 Bake in the preheated oven for about 45 minutes, until the fruit is cooked and the topping is golden brown.
6 Serve hot or cold with home-made custard or yogurt.

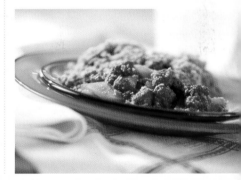

sensuous *foods*

EATING CAN BE A *sensuous experience and some foods even seem to arouse sensual feelings. The recipes in this section can help lift the spirits and increase alertness. Foods such as apricots,* bananas, *avocado, green leafy and root vegetables, legumes, nuts, eggs, poultry, oily fish, chicken liver, and kidneys are good sources of B group vitamins that can affect the way we feel.*

goat cheese *and* spinach salad

This tasty salad is quick and easy to prepare and makes an ideal appetizer or snack. Protein foods such as goat cheese can be stimulating and mentally arousing, and some people say they help lift moods.

ingredients

- 4 ounces (115g) baby spinach
- 2 ounces (55g) watercress
- ½ cup/1 ounce (25g) alfalfa sprouts
- 1 cup/4 ounces (115g) chopped sugar-snap peas (mangetout)
- 9 ounces (250g) cherry tomatoes, halved
- 4tbsp French dressing (see recipe on page 21)
- sea salt
- freshly ground black pepper
- 8 ounces (225g) goat cheese, thinly sliced or diced

serves *four*
preparation time *10 minutes*

method

1 Put the spinach, watercress, alfalfa sprouts, sugar-snap peas, and tomatoes in a bowl and toss together.
2 Whisk the dressing to ensure it is well mixed and adjust the seasoning if necessary. Drizzle over the salad vegetables and toss.
3 Divide the salad among four plates and scatter some goat cheese over the top.
4 Serve immediately with whole-wheat bread.

variations

- *Use shredded round (butterhead) lettuce leaves instead of watercress.*
- *Use arugula instead of alfalfa sprouts.*

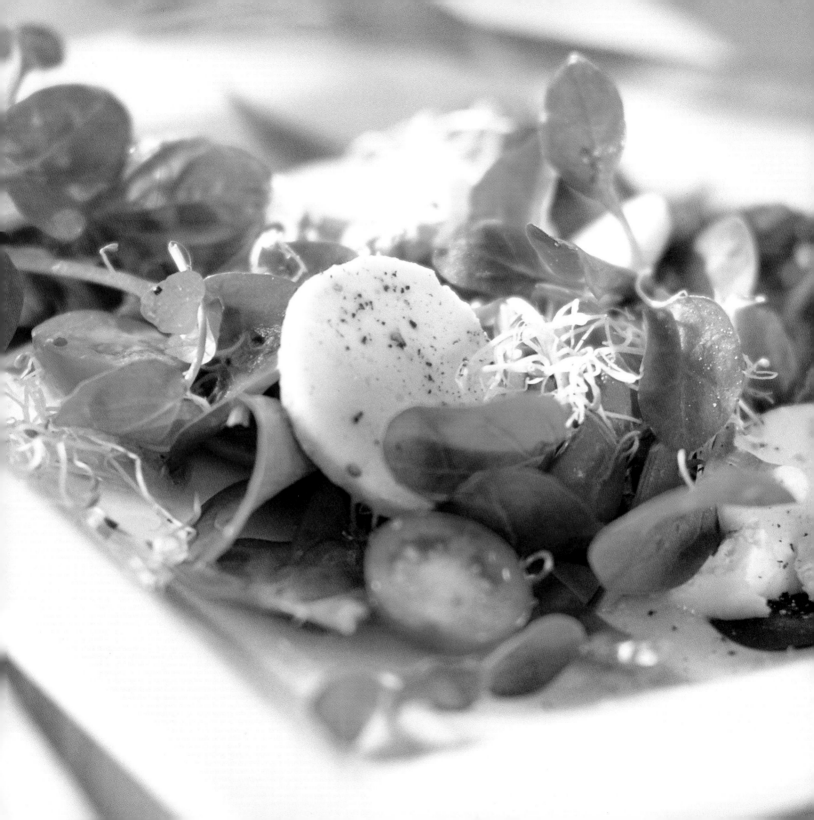

fresh mushroom soup

This fresh mushroom soup is a delicious and warming appetizer. Mushrooms and parsley contain B vitamins and iron. Deficiencies of these nutrients can result in impaired brain function.

■ ingredients

- 2 tbsp/1 ounce (25g) butter
- 1 onion, chopped
- 12 ounces (350g) cremini mushrooms, sliced
- 1¼ cups/½ pint (300ml) vegetable stock (see recipe on page 20)
- 1¼ cups/½ pint (300ml) milk
- sea salt
- freshly ground black pepper
- 1–2tbsp chopped fresh parsley
- fresh parsley sprigs, to garnish

serves *four*
preparation time *10 minutes*
cooking time *25–30 minutes*

■ method

1 Melt the butter in a large saucepan. Add the onion and cook gently for 3 minutes.
2 Add the mushrooms and cook gently for 5 minutes.
3 Stir in the stock, milk, and seasoning; then cover and bring to a boil. Reduce the heat and simmer for 15–20 minutes, stirring occasionally, until the vegetables are cooked and tender.
4 Remove the pan from the heat and let cool slightly; then blend in a food processor.
5 Return the soup to the rinsed-out saucepan. Stir in the chopped parsley and reheat gently until piping hot, stirring occasionally.
6 Ladle into warmed soup bowls. Garnish with the parsley sprigs and serve with whole-wheat rolls.

variations

· *Use regular or button mushrooms instead of cremini mushrooms.*
· *Use 2 leeks instead of the onion.*

chicken *and* asparagus frittata

A great alternative to an omelet, this appetizing frittata makes an ideal first course or main dish. Chicken and eggs are both good sources of high-quality protein.

■ ingredients

- 4 ounces (115g) asparagus tips
- 2tbsp olive oil
- 4 ounces (115g) zucchini, thinly sliced
- 1 bunch green onions, chopped
- 6 medium eggs
- 1 7-ounce (200g) can corn kernels, drained
- 1¾ cups/8 ounces (225g) diced, cooked skinless, boneless chicken breast
- ½ cup/2 ounces (55g) grated Cheddar cheese
- 1tbsp chopped fresh parsley
- 1tbsp chopped fresh tarragon
- sea salt
- freshly ground black pepper
- fresh herb sprigs, to garnish

serves *four to six*
preparation time *10 minutes*
cooking time *25–30 minutes*

■ method

1 Cook the asparagus in boiling water for 4 minutes. Drain well and keep warm.
2 Heat the oil in a large nonstick skillet. Add the zucchini and green onions, and cook gently for 5 minutes.
3 Beat the eggs in a bowl; then stir in the asparagus, corn, chicken, cheese, herbs, and seasoning. Pour the egg mixture into the skillet and stir briefly, spreading the mixture out evenly.
4 Cook until the eggs are beginning to set and the frittata is golden brown underneath.
5 Preheat the broiler to medium. Broil the frittata until the top is golden brown.
6 Cut into wedges and garnish with the herb sprigs. Serve hot with a mixed dark-green leaf side salad.

variations

· *Use mushrooms instead of zucchini.*
· *Use cooked turkey, tuna, or salmon instead of chicken.*

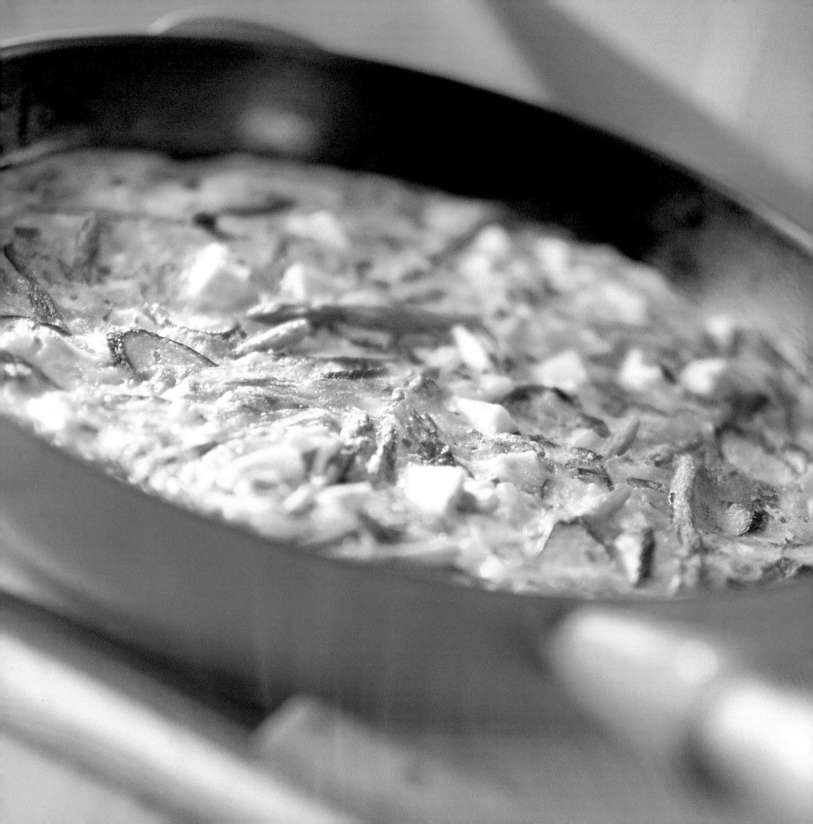

tuna *and* shrimp savory pie

This seafood pie makes a nutritious meal served with baked potatoes and a mixed salad. Fish and shellfish contain an amino acid called tyrosine, which is used to make brain-stimulating chemicals that increase mental energy and alertness.

ingredients

for the pastry

- 1¼ cups/5 ounces (140g) whole-wheat flour
- ¼ cup/1 ounce (25g) uncooked oatmeal
- dash of salt
- ⅓ cup/3 ounces (85g) butter, chopped

for the filling

- 1 14-ounce (100g) can tuna in water, drained and flaked
- 1 cup/4 ounces (115g) small cooked, shelled shrimp
- ½ cup/4 ounces (115g) drained, canned corn kernels
- 1 tomato, skinned and chopped
- 2 medium eggs
- ⅔ cup/¼ pint (150ml) milk
- ½ cup/2 ounces (55g) finely grated Cheddar cheese
- 1–2tbsp chopped fresh basil
- sea salt
- freshly ground black pepper
- fresh herb sprigs, to garnish

serves *four to six*
preparation time *15 minutes, plus 20 minutes chilling time*
cooking time *55 minutes*

method

1 Preheat the oven to 400°F.
2 To make the pastry, put the flour, oatmeal, and salt in a bowl; then lightly rub in the butter until the mixture resembles bread crumbs. Add enough cold water to form a soft dough.
3 Roll the dough out on a lightly floured surface and use to line an 8-inch (20cm) pie pan. Cover and chill for 20 minutes.
4 Line the pie shell with nonstick baking parchment and fill with baking beans. Place on a baking tray and bake blind for about 10 minutes, until firm and lightly brown. Remove from the oven and lift out the paper and beans.
5 Reduce the oven temperature to 350°F.
6 Mix the tuna, shrimp, and corn together. Spoon into the pie shell. Scatter with chopped tomato.
7 Beat the eggs, milk, cheese, basil, and seasoning, and pour into the pie shell.

8 Bake for about 45 minutes, until risen, lightly set and golden brown.
9 Garnish with the herb sprigs and serve warm or cold in slices with baked potatoes and a mixed side salad.

variations

- *Use canned salmon and cooked mussels instead of tuna and shrimp.*
- *Use chopped fresh chives or parsley instead of basil.*

freezing instructions

Let cool completely, then wrap in foil or seal in a freezer bag and label. Freeze for up to 3 months. Defrost for several hours, or overnight in the refrigerator. Serve cold or reheat in a moderate oven.

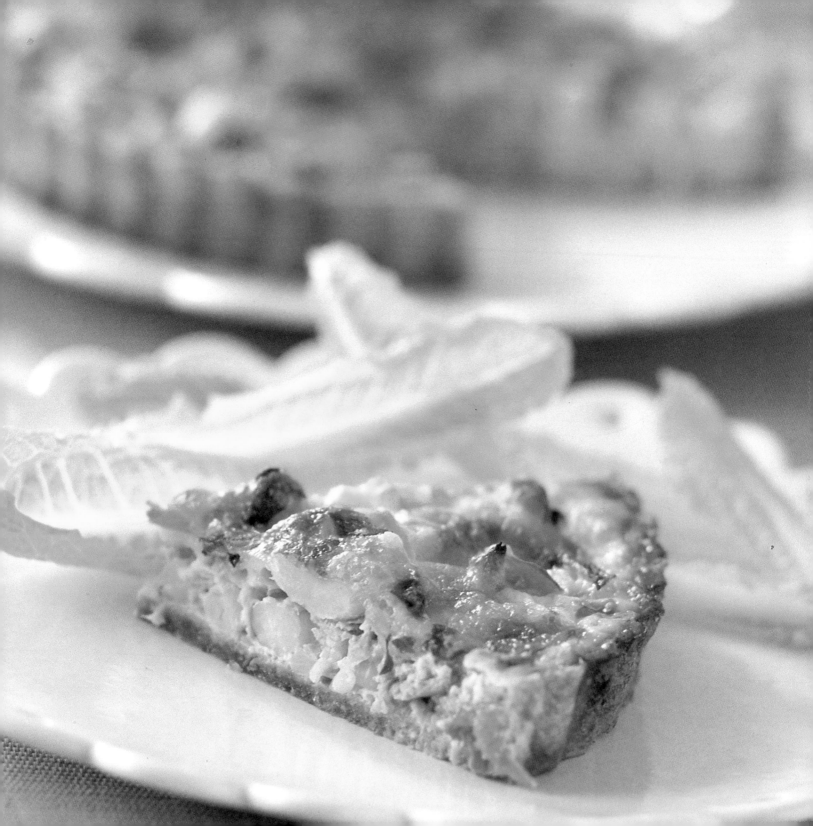

broiled lemon sole *with* fresh parsley sauce

 Fresh lemon sole is a good source of protein, magnesium, selenium, and B vitamins, all of which are important brain nutrients.

ingredients

- 2tbsp cornstarch
- 1¼ cups/½ pint (300ml) milk
- 2–3tbsp chopped fresh parsley
- 1 tbsp/½ ounce (15g) butter
- sea salt
- freshly ground black pepper
- 8 lemon sole fillets
- 2tbsp olive oil
- fresh parsley sprigs, to garnish

serves *four*
preparation time *10 minutes*
cooking time *4–6 minutes*

method

1 Line a broiler rack with foil.
2 In a saucepan, blend the cornstarch with a little of the milk. Stir in the remaining milk; then heat gently, stirring continuously, until the sauce comes to a boil and thickens. Simmer gently for 2 minutes, stirring.
3 Add the chopped parsley, butter, and seasoning, and heat gently until piping hot, stirring continuously. Keep the sauce hot while cooking the fish.
4 Place the lemon sole fillets on the broiler rack and brush lightly with oil. Broil for 4–6 minutes, until the fish is cooked and the flesh just flakes when tested with a fork, carefully turning the fillets over once during cooking.

5 Place two cooked fish fillets on each warmed serving plate. Pour some parsley sauce over the fish and garnish with parsley sprigs.
6 Serve with cooked fresh vegetables such as new potatoes, baby carrots, and broccoli.

variations

- *Serve the parsley sauce with other cooked white fish.*
- *Use fresh chives instead of parsley.*

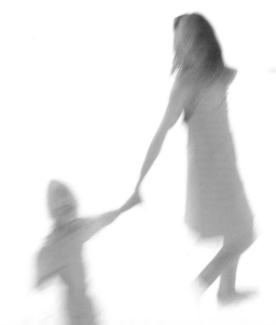

fish *dishes*

turkey breasts *with* cranberry sauce

 Cranberry sauce is a traditional and delicious accompaniment to turkey. Turkey breasts are especially high in protein.

ingredients

- 2½ cups/8 ounces (225g) fresh, frozen (defrosted) or canned (drained) cranberries
- I eating apple, peeled, cored, and finely chopped
- ¾ cup/6 ounces (175g) light brown sugar
- I–2tbsp port
- a little olive oil, for brushing
- 6 turkey breasts, each about 4½ ounces (125g)
- sea salt
- freshly ground black pepper
- fresh herb sprigs, to garnish

serves *six*
preparation time *20 minutes*
cooking time *20 minutes*

method

I To make the sauce, put the cranberries and chopped apple in a saucepan with ⅔ cup/¼ pint (150ml) water. Cover and bring to a boil; then reduce the heat and simmer for about 10 minutes, until the fruit is soft. If using canned cranberries, they need only be warmed through.

2 Stir in the sugar (canned cranberries will need a little extra), then cook gently until the sugar has dissolved, stirring constantly. Stir in the port and remove the pan from the heat.

3 Preheat the broiler to medium. Lightly brush the turkey breasts with oil and season with salt and pepper. Place the turkey breasts on a broiler rack in a broiler pan and broil for about 20 minutes, until cooked and tender, turning once.

4 Serve the turkey with warm or cold cranberry sauce spooned alongside.

5 Garnish with the herb sprigs and serve with oven-baked fresh vegetables and brown rice.

variations

- Use brandy or sherry instead of port.
- Use I pear instead of the apple.

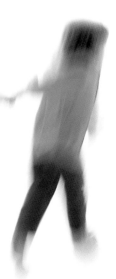

lamb *and* vegetable couscous

 This casserole of lamb and vegetables served on a bed of hot couscous will be popular with the whole family. Lamb is high in protein, iron, and B vitamins. The complex carbohydrates in couscous may increase the level of serotonin, a brain chemical that helps you feel calmer and more relaxed.

ingredients

- 1 tbsp olive oil
- 12 ounces (350g) lean lamb fillet, cut into 1-inch (2.5cm) cubes
- 1 onion, sliced
- 1 large clove garlic, chopped
- 1 green bell pepper, seeded and sliced
- 3 celery stalks, chopped
- 3 carrots, thinly sliced
- 8 ounces (225g) baby new potatoes
- 1 tsp each ground cumin, ground coriander, and hot chili powder
- 1 14-ounce (400g) can tomatoes, chopped
- ⅔ cup/¼ pint (150ml) vegetable stock (see recipe on page 20)
- sea salt and black pepper
- 6 ounces (175g) cauliflower florets
- 2 cups/12 ounces (350g) couscous
- 2 tbsp/1 ounce (25g) butter
- fresh herb sprigs, to garnish

serves *four*
preparation time *15 minutes*
cooking time *about 1 hour*

method

1 Heat the oil in a large saucepan. Add the lamb and cook until brown all over, stirring occasionally.
2 Add the onion and garlic, and cook gently for 3 minutes.
3 Add the green pepper, celery, carrots, new potatoes, and ground spices, and cook for 1 minute, stirring.
4 Stir in the tomatoes, stock, and seasoning. Cover and bring to a boil; reduce the heat and simmer for 30 minutes, stirring occasionally.
5 Stir in the cauliflower; then cover and simmer for another 30–45 minutes, until the lamb and vegetables are cooked and tender, stirring occasionally.
6 Meanwhile, cook the couscous according to the directions on the package.
7 Stir the butter into the hot couscous; then spoon it onto warmed serving plates. Spoon the lamb and vegetables on top and serve hot, garnished with fresh herb sprigs.

variations

- *Thicken the sauce with a little cornstarch before serving. Blend 1 tbsp cornstarch with 2tbsp water. Stir into the cooked lamb and vegetable sauce, and bring to a boil, stirring continuously. Simmer gently for 2 minutes, stirring, then serve.*
- *Use skinless, boneless chicken or turkey instead of lamb.*
- *Use parsnips instead of carrots.*

freezing instructions

The sauce can be frozen. Let cool completely, then transfer to a rigid, freezeproof container. Cover, seal, and label. Freeze for up to 3 months. Defrost for several hours, or overnight in the refrigerator. Reheat gently in a saucepan until hot.

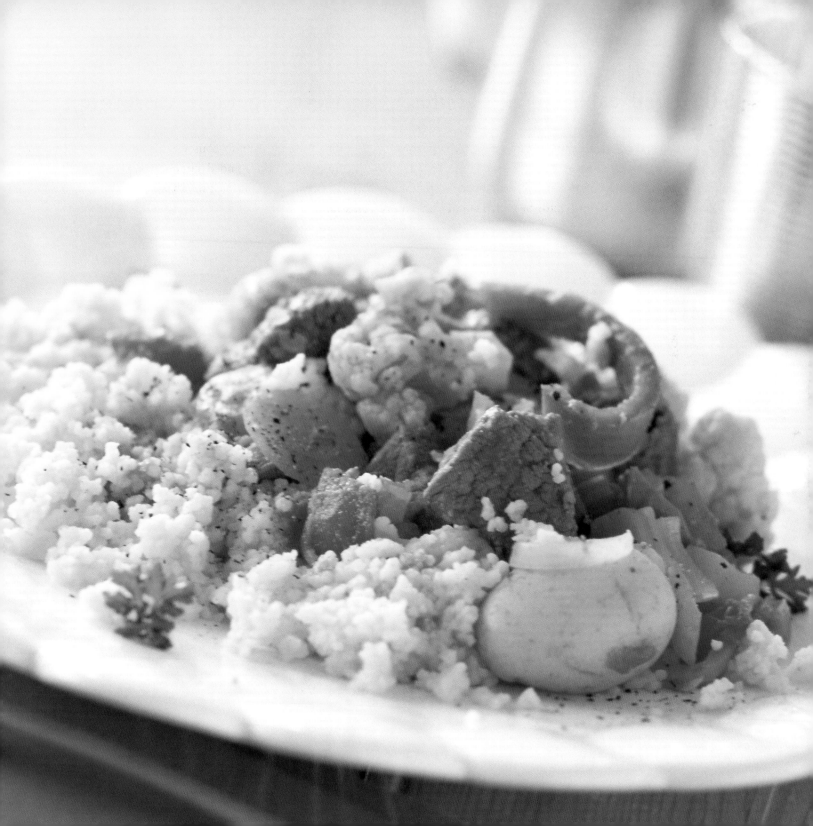

baked red cabbage *with* apples

Oven-baked red cabbage can be served with baked potatoes and cheese—or it makes a delicious accompaniment to grilled lean meat or fish. Cabbage is a good source of vitamin C and some of the B vitamins.

■ ingredients

- 1 pound (450g) shredded red cabbage
- 2 eating apples, peeled, cored, and sliced
- 6 shallots (French shallots), thinly sliced
- 1 clove garlic, crushed
- 2tbsp unsweetened apple juice
- 2tsp honey
- 2tsp red wine vinegar
- sea salt
- freshly ground black pepper
- 1 tbsp/½ ounce (15g) butter
- ¼–⅓ cup/1–2 ounces (25–55g) toasted pine nuts (optional)
- fresh herb sprigs, to garnish

serves *four as an accompaniment*
preparation time *10 minutes*
cooking time *1–1½ hours*

■ method

1 Preheat the oven to 375°F.
2 Put the cabbage, apples, shallots, garlic, apple juice, honey, vinegar, and seasoning in an ovenproof casserole and mix well. Cover and bake for 1–1½ hours, until the vegetables are cooked and tender, stirring once or twice.
3 Stir in the butter and pine nuts, if using, and serve hot, garnished with the herb sprigs.
4 Serve with oven-baked potatoes topped with a little grated Cheddar cheese or diced goat cheese.

variations

- *Use 1 onion instead of shallots.*
- *Use unsweetened grape juice or medium cider instead of apple juice.*
- *Use flaked or chopped almonds instead of pine nuts.*

harvest vegetable casserole

This nutritious and warming vegetable casserole makes a delicious dish for chilly winter evenings. Fresh vegetables are a good source of B vitamins and vitamin C, which are good for the brain and nervous system.

■ ingredients

- 1 pound (450g) potatoes, thinly sliced
- 2tbsp olive oil
- 8 ounces (225g) pearl onions or shallots (French shallots)
- 1 clove garlic, crushed
- 2 celery stalks, chopped
- 8 ounces (225g) carrots, thinly sliced
- 1¾ cups/8 ounces (225g) diced rutabaga
- 1¾ cups/8 ounces (225g) diced parsnips
- 1¾ cups/8 ounces (225g) small cauliflower florets
- 1 14-ounce (400g) can tomatoes, chopped
- 1¼ cups/½ pint (300ml) vegetable stock (see recipe on page 20)
- ⅔ cup/¼ pint (150ml) dry white wine
- 2tsp dried *herbes de provence*
- sea salt
- freshly ground black pepper
- 1tbsp cornstarch
- fresh herb sprigs, to garnish

serves *four to six*
preparation time *30 minutes*
cooking time *1 hour*

■ method

1 Preheat the oven to 400°F.
2 Parboil the potatoes in boiling water, then drain. Toss in 1 tbsp oil.
3 Heat the remaining oil in a large saucepan. Add the onions or shallots, garlic, and celery, and cook for 3 minutes, stirring constantly.
4 Add the carrots, rutabaga, vegetables, stock, wine, dried herbs, and seasoning, and mix well.
5 Blend the cornstarch with 2tbsp water and stir into the vegetables. Bring to a boil, stirring until the mixture thickens.
6 Transfer the vegetables to an ovenproof dish. Arrange the potato slices over the top, Cover with foil and bake for about 1 hour, until tender. Remove the foil for the last 20 minutes.
7 Garnish with the herb sprigs.

variation

- *Use celeriac instead of rutabaga.*

vegetable *dishes*

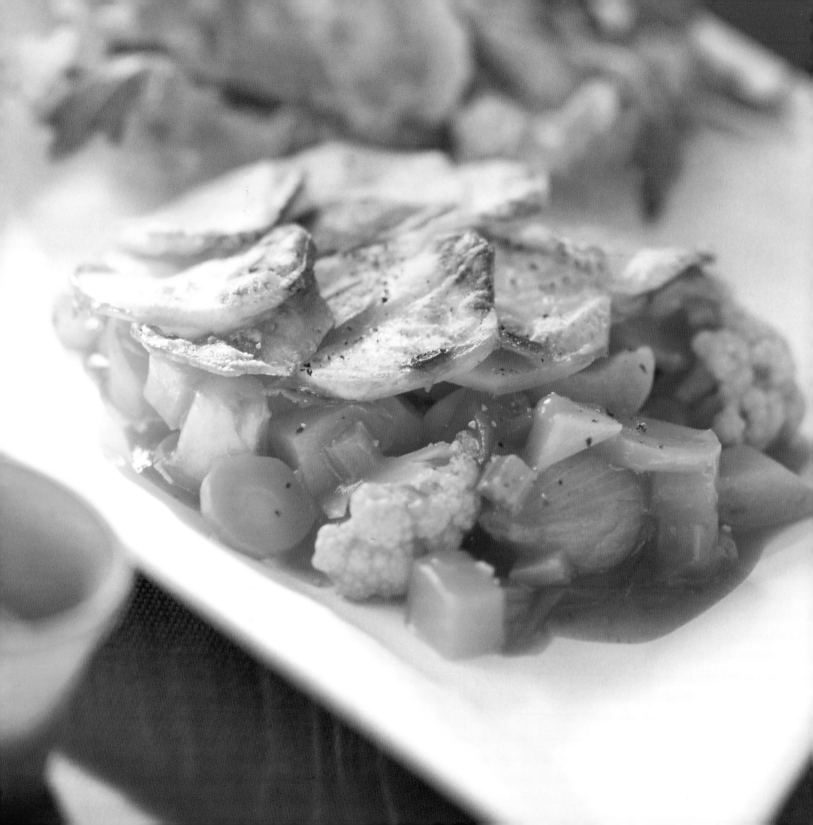

curried tofu *and* broad bean salad

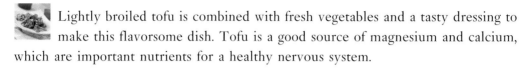 Lightly broiled tofu is combined with fresh vegetables and a tasty dressing to make this flavorsome dish. Tofu is a good source of magnesium and calcium, which are important nutrients for a healthy nervous system.

ingredients

- 12 ounces (350g) tofu, cut into 1-inch (2.5cm) cubes
- 3tbsp olive oil
- 1½tsp ground coriander
- 1½tsp ground cumin
- 1tsp hot chili powder
- 1tsp ground turmeric
- sea salt
- freshly ground black pepper
- 1⅓ cups/8 ounces (225g) frozen broad beans
- 1⅓ cups/8 ounces (225g) green beans, cut into 2-inch (5cm) lengths
- 2 cups/4 ounces (115g) shredded round (butterhead) lettuce
- 1 bunch green onions, chopped

for the dressing
- 6tbsp tomato juice
- 2tsp balsamic vinegar
- 1tsp Dijon mustard
- 1 clove garlic, crushed
- 1 tbsp (15ml) chopped fresh basil

serves *four*
preparation time *25 minutes, plus 30 minutes marinating time*
cooking time *6–8 minutes*

method

1 Thread the tofu pieces onto long skewers.

2 In a small bowl, mix together the oil, ground spices, and seasoning. Brush the oil mixture all over the tofu. Place the skewers on a plate, cover, and set aside for 30 minutes.

3 Cook the broad beans and green beans in a saucepan of boiling water for 4–5 minutes, until tender. Drain and rinse under cold running water; then drain thoroughly and set aside to cool.

4 Put the lettuce and green onions in a bowl. Add the cooled beans and toss.

5 Put the tomato juice, vinegar, mustard, garlic, basil, and seasoning in a small bowl and whisk until thoroughly mixed.

6 Drizzle the dressing over the salad and toss together. Set aside.

7 Preheat the broiler to high. Place the tofu skewers on a broiler rack in a broiler pan and broil for 3–4 minutes on each side, until lightly browned.

8 Remove the tofu from the skewers and add to the bean salad; toss lightly.

9 Serve immediately with crispbread or crusty whole-wheat bread.

variations
- *Use 1–2tbsp curry powder or curry paste instead of ground spices.*
- *Use canned (drained) corn kernels instead of green beans. Do not cook the corn.*

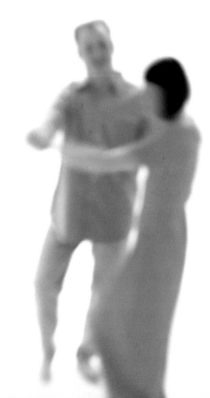

vegetable *dishes*

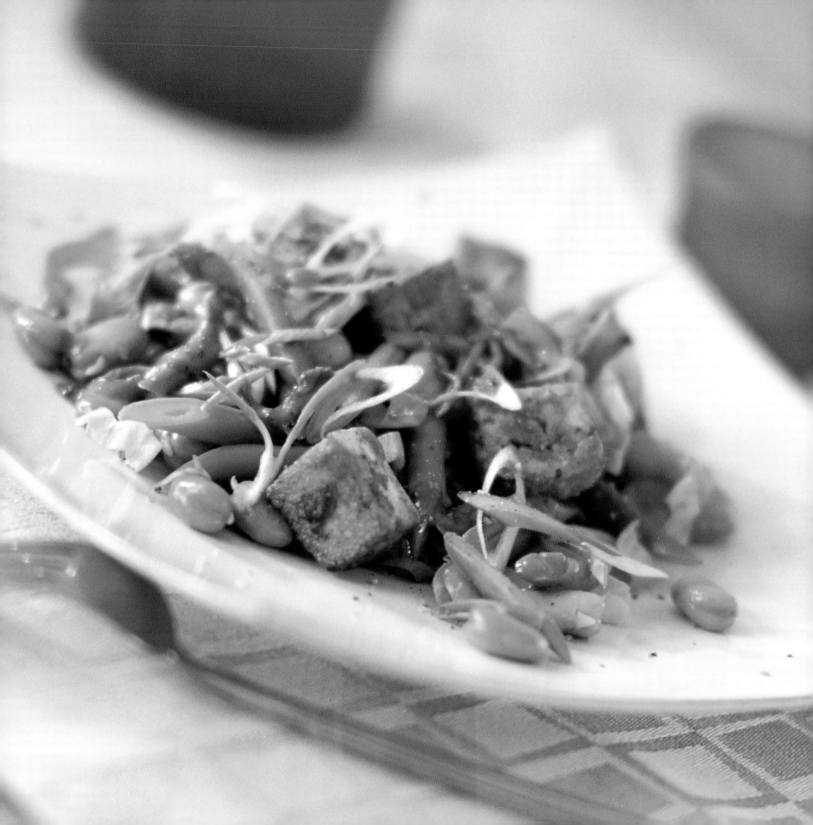

hazelnut meringues

These meringues, sandwiched together with crème fraîche or whipped cream, make an irresistible dessert. Hazelnuts contain B vitamins, boron, and iron.

■ ingredients

- 3 medium egg whites
- ¾ cup/6 ounces (175g) light brown sugar
- ½ cup/2 ounces (55g) toasted hazelnuts, ground or finely chopped
- ½tsp ground cinnamon
- ⅔ cup/5 ounces (150g) crème fraîche or whipped cream
- 8 ounces (225g) small strawberries, halved
- 2 kiwi fruit, peeled and sliced
- fresh mint sprigs, to decorate

serves *four* (*makes 8 pairs of meringues*)
preparation time *20 minutes*
cooking time *2–3 hours*

■ method

1 Preheat the oven to 225°F.
2 Line two baking trays with nonstick baking paper.
3 Put the egg whites in a bowl and whisk until stiff. Gradually whisk in the sugar, until the egg whites are stiff and shiny.
4 Gently fold in the hazelnuts and ground cinnamon.
5 Spoon the meringue mixture onto the baking trays to make 16 small mounds. Bake for 2–3 hours until firm and crisp. Transfer to a wire rack to cool; then carefully peel off the paper.
6 Sandwich pairs of meringues with the crème fraîche or whipped cream.
7 Serve at once with strawberry halves and kiwi slices. Decorate with the mint sprigs.

variations

• *Use almonds instead of hazelnuts.*
• *Use a few drops of vanilla or almond extract instead of cinnamon.*

peach *and* banana cream

This delicious cream is ideal for a quick and nutritious family dessert. Yogurt is a protein food, containing chemicals to stimulate and arouse the mind. Bananas are a good source of vitamin B_6.

■ ingredients

- 1 14-ounce (410g) can peaches in fruit juice, drained
- 2 bananas, peeled, sliced, and tossed in a little lemon juice
- 2tbsp honey
- 1tsp ground ginger
- 1 cup/9 ounces (250g) plain yogurt
- ⅔ cup/5 ounces (140g) crème fraîche or whipped cream
- ¼ cup/1 ounce (25g) toasted flaked almonds, to decorate

serves *six*
preparation time *10 minutes, plus 30 minutes chilling time*

■ method

1 Put the peaches, bananas, honey, and ginger in a blender or food processor and blend until smooth. Transfer the mixture to a bowl.
2 Fold the yogurt and crème fraîche or whipped cream into the fruit mixture, mixing well.
3 Spoon into serving glasses or dishes and refrigerate for 30 minutes before serving.
4 Sprinkle flaked almonds over the top before serving.
5 Serve with homemade oat or whole-wheat cookies.

variations

• *Use canned apricots or pears instead of peaches.*
• *Use ground cinnamon or nutmeg instead of ginger.*

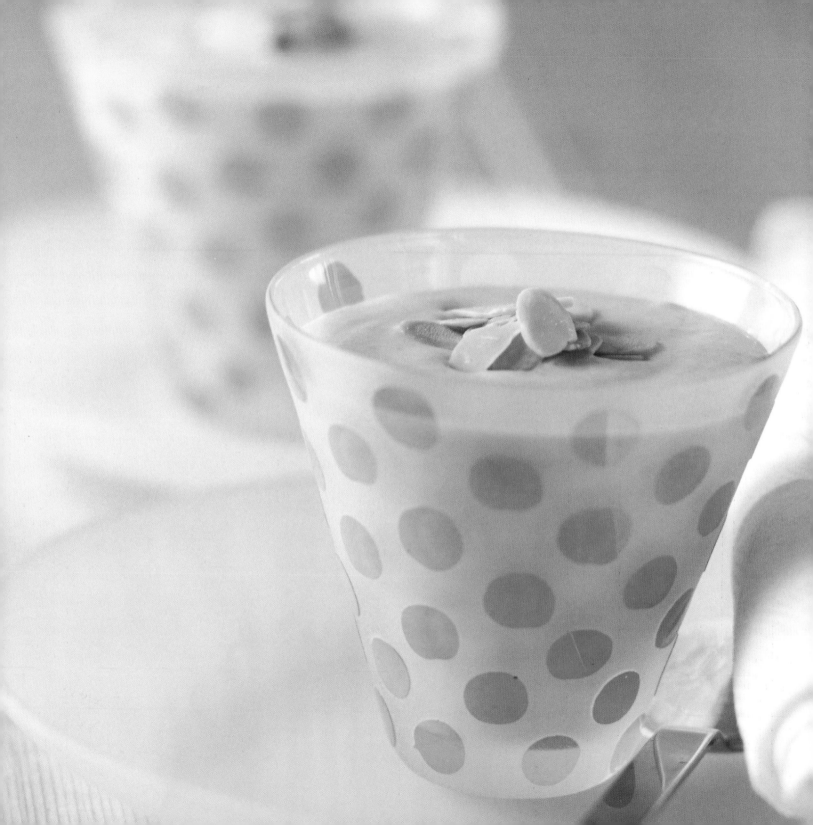

fruity florentines

These florentines made of mixed fruit, nuts, and seeds are wonderful for a packed lunch or snack. Chocolate can be wonderfully calming and soothing, and makes us feel good.

ingredients

- ¼ cup/2 ounces (55g) butter
- ¼ cup/2 ounces (55g light brown sugar
- 1tbsp maple syrup
- ¼ cup/1 ounce (25g) whole-wheat flour
- ½ cup/3 ounces (85g) mixed dried fruit, including golden raisins, raisins, and chopped, ready-to-eat dried apricots
- ½ cup/2 ounces (55g) roughly chopped mixed nuts, including walnuts, hazelnuts, and almonds
- 3tbsp/1 ounce (25g) mixed sunflower and pumpkin seeds
- 4 squares/4 ounces (115g) dark chocolate, broken into pieces

makes *12–14*
preparation time *20 minutes*
cooking time *10–15 minutes*

method

1 Preheat the oven to 325°F.
2 Line two large baking trays with nonstick baking paper.
3 Put the butter, sugar, and syrup in a saucepan and heat gently until melted, stirring constantly.
4 Remove the pan from the heat; then stir in the flour, dried fruit, nuts, and seeds.
5 Drop teaspoonfuls of the mixture onto the baking trays, allowing room between each one for spreading.
6 Bake for 10–15 minutes, until golden brown. Remove from the oven and immediately push in the edges of the florentines with a nonstick spatula to neaten the round shapes. Leave on the baking sheets for a few minutes to firm up slightly; then transfer to a wire rack to cool completely.
7 Put the chocolate in a bowl over a saucepan of simmering water and stir until melted. Remove from the heat.
8 Spread some chocolate over the smooth side of each florentine; then place on a wire rack, chocolate-side up, and let set completely before serving.

variations

• For a delicious dessert, serve the florentines with fresh fruit, such as strawberries and raspberries, and a little plain yogurt.
• Use honey instead of maple syrup.

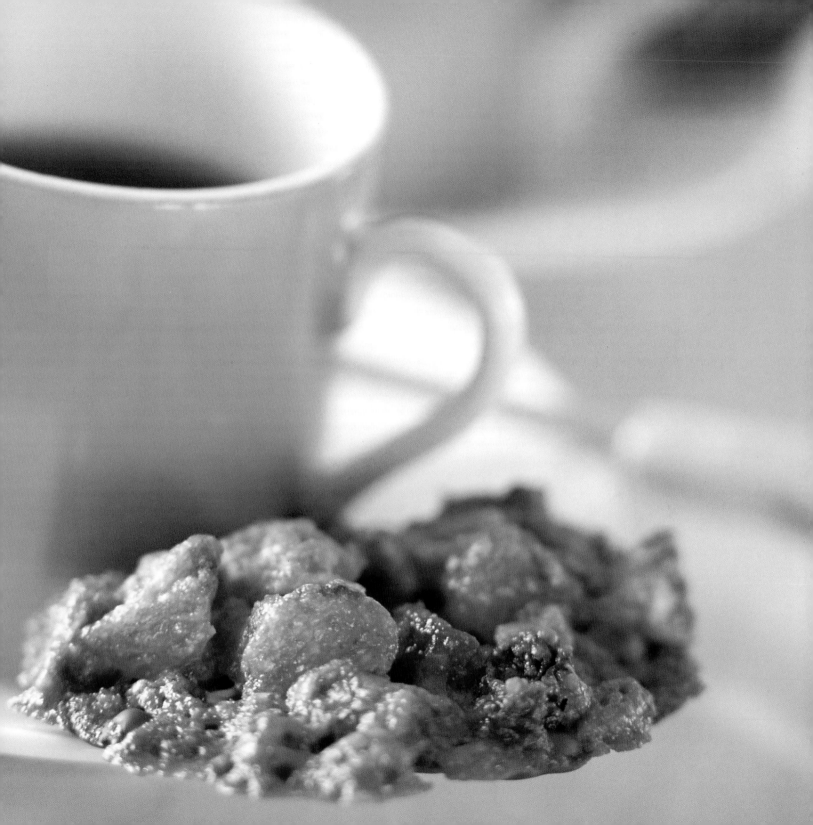

dinner for two

SMOOTH AWAY YOUR *lover's furrowed brow and get into a relaxing, seductive mood with this deliciously arousing menu. These recipes will* provide you with enough energy for a night of passion. The protein and carbohydrates will help to increase the level of soothing hormones.*

goat cheese *and* spinach salad

This sensuous salad could help chase away the blues and lighten your mood.

■ ingredients

- 4 ounces (115g) baby spinach
- 2 ounces (55g) watercress
- ½ cup/1 ounce (25g) alfalfa sprouts
- 1 cup/4 ounces (115g) chopped sugar-snap peas (mangetout)
- 9 ounces (250g) cherry tomatoes, halved
- 4tbsp French dressing (see recipe on page 21)
- sea salt
- freshly ground black pepper
- 8 ounces (225g) goat cheese, thinly sliced or diced

serves *four*
preparation time *10 minutes*

■ method

1 Put the spinach, watercress, alfalfa sprouts, sugar-snap peas, and tomatoes in a bowl and toss together.
2 Whisk the dressing to ensure it is well mixed and adjust the seasoning if necessary. Drizzle over the salad vegetables and toss.
3 Divide the salad among four plates and scatter some goat cheese over the top.
4 Serve immediately with whole-wheat bread.

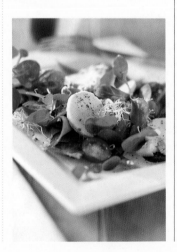

lamb *and* vegetable couscous

Lamb provides the mentally arousing protein and the complex carbohydrates in the couscous help to increase the brain's level of soothing serotonin.

■ ingredients

- 1tbsp olive oil
- 12 ounces (350g) lean lamb fillet, cut into 1-inch (2.5cm) cubes
- 1 onion, sliced
- 1 large clove garlic, chopped
- 1 green bell pepper, seeded and sliced
- 3 celery stalks, chopped
- 3 carrots, thinly sliced
- 8 ounces (225g) baby new potatoes
- 1tsp each ground cumin, ground coriander, and hot chili powder
- 1 14-ounce (400g) can tomatoes, chopped
- ⅔ cup/¼ pint (150ml) vegetable stock (see recipe on page 20)
- sea salt and black pepper
- 6 ounces (175g) cauliflower florets
- 2 cups/12 ounces (350g) couscous
- 2 tbsp/1 ounce (25g) butter
- fresh herb sprigs, to garnish

serves *four*
preparation time *15 minutes*
cooking time *about 1 hour*

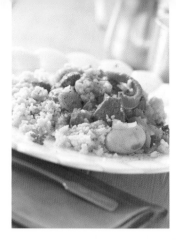

method

1 Heat the oil in a large saucepan. Add the lamb and cook until brown all over, stirring occasionally.

2 Add the onion and garlic, and cook gently for 3 minutes.

3 Add the green pepper, celery, carrots, new potatoes, and ground spices, and cook for 1 minute, stirring.

4 Stir in the tomatoes, stock, and seasoning. Cover and bring to a boil; reduce the heat and simmer for 30 minutes, stirring occasionally.

5 Stir in the cauliflower; then cover and simmer for another 30–45 minutes, until the lamb and vegetables are cooked and tender, stirring occasionally.

6 Meanwhile, cook the couscous according to the directions on the package.

7 Stir the butter into the hot couscous; then spoon it onto warmed serving plates. Spoon the lamb and vegetables on top and serve hot, garnished with fresh herb sprigs.

peach *and* banana cream

The yogurt in this cream contains tryptophan to soothe and arouse a tired mind.

ingredients

- 1 14-ounce (410g) can peaches in fruit juice, drained
- 2 bananas, peeled, sliced, and tossed in a little lemon juice
- 2tbsp honey
- 1tsp ground ginger
- 1 cup/9 ounces (250g) plain yogurt
- ⅔ cup/5 ounces (140g) crème fraîche or whipped cream
- ¼ cup/1 ounce (25g) toasted flaked almonds, to decorate

serves *six*
preparation time *10 minutes, plus 30 minutes chilling time*

method

1 Put the peaches, bananas, honey, and ginger in a blender or food processor and blend until smooth. Transfer the mixture to a bowl.

2 Fold the yogurt and crème fraîche or whipped cream into the fruit mixture, mixing well.

3 Spoon into serving glasses or dishes and refrigerate for 30 minutes before serving.

4 Sprinkle flaked almonds over the top before serving.

5 Serve with homemade oat or whole-wheat cookies.

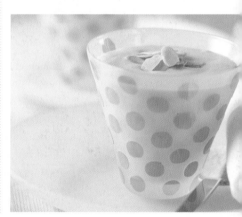

feel-good *foods*

IF YOU NEED *to be wide awake, and in top form, eat protein foods as part of a balanced meal for breakfast and lunch. Scrambled eggs, omelets, yogurt, cheese, fresh fish, all kinds of beans, chicken, and lean meat are all first-class protein providers.*

Extra supplies of vitamin C are important when it comes to helping the body cope when under stress. Nearly all fruits and vegetables contain some vitamin C, but good sources are citrus fruit, apricots, bell peppers, kiwi fruit, and green leafy vegetables.

mixed leaf *and* toasted nut salad

This simple salad is quick to prepare and makes a nutritious appetizer or snack. Almonds and hazelnuts supply B vitamins, magnesium, iron, and essential fatty acids, all of which are important for a healthy brain and nervous system.

ingredients

- ½ cup/2 ounces (55g) whole blanched hazelnuts
- ½ cup/2 ounces (55g) whole blanched almonds
- ½ cup/2 ounces (55g) pine nuts
- 4 ounces (125g) mixed salad leaves such as lollo rosso (coral lettuce), watercress, and spinach
- 2 ounces (55g) arugula
- 1 cup/4 ounces (115g) chopped sugar-snap peas (mangetout)
- 6tbsp French dressing (see recipe on page 21)

serves *four*
preparation time *15 minutes*
cooking time *3–5 minutes*

method

1 Preheat the broiler to medium. Spread the hazelnuts, almonds, and pine nuts out on a baking tray. Broil for a few minutes, turning frequently, until lightly browned. Cool; then chop roughly.
2 Put the salad leaves, arugula, and sugar-snap peas in a large bowl and toss. Divide the salad among four serving plates or bowls and scatter some nuts over each salad.
3 Drizzle a little dressing over each salad. Toss lightly and serve with whole-wheat bread.

variations

- *Use walnuts and cashew nuts instead of hazelnuts and almonds.*
- *Use arugula instead of watercress.*
- *Whisk 1tsp of finely grated lemon rind into the French dressing before serving.*

soups *and* appetizers

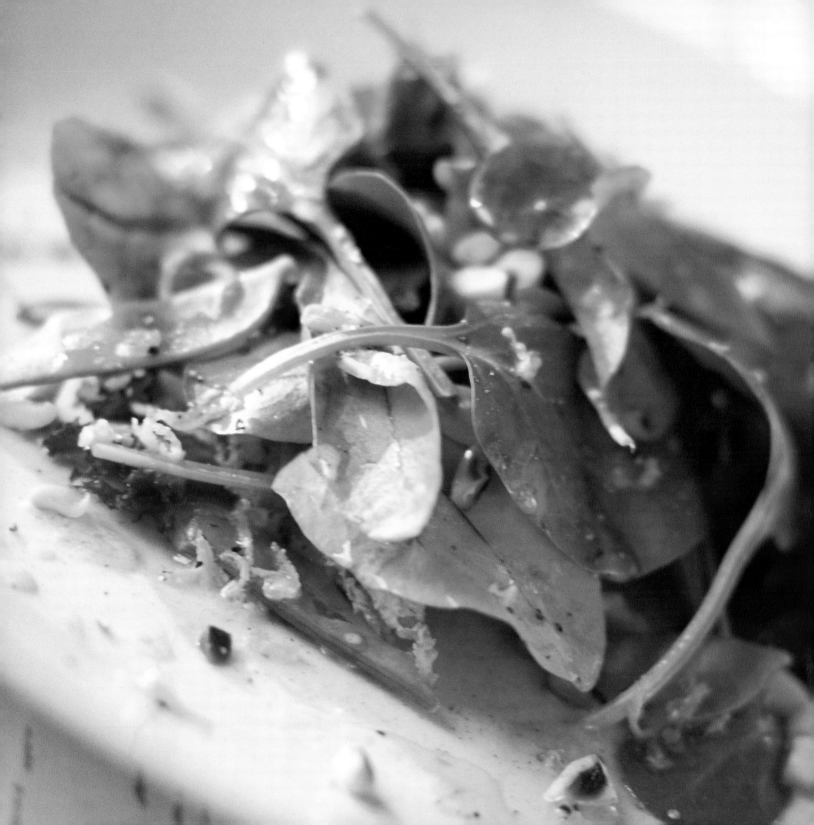

pink grapefruit *with* cinnamon

Juicy grapefruit, sprinkled with a little sugar and cinnamon and lightly broiled, makes a refreshing appetizer. Fresh fruit is a good source of vitamin C, an anti-stress nutrient that helps to lift moods.

ingredients

- 2 pink grapefruit
- 2tbsp light brown sugar
- 1–2tsp ground cinnamon
- fresh mint sprigs, to garnish (optional)

serves *four*
preparation time *10 minutes*
cooking time *3–5 minutes*

method

1 Preheat the broiler to medium. Cut each grapefruit in half; then cut between the segments to loosen the flesh.
2 Mix the sugar and cinnamon together and sprinkle over the grapefruit.
3 Place the grapefruit on a broiler rack in a broiler pan and broil for a few minutes, until the sugar has melted and the grapefruit are hot.
4 Serve immediately, garnished with the mint sprigs, if you like.

variations

- *Use regular white grapefruit instead of pink grapefruit.*
- *Use ginger instead of cinnamon.*
- *Use honey instead of sugar.*

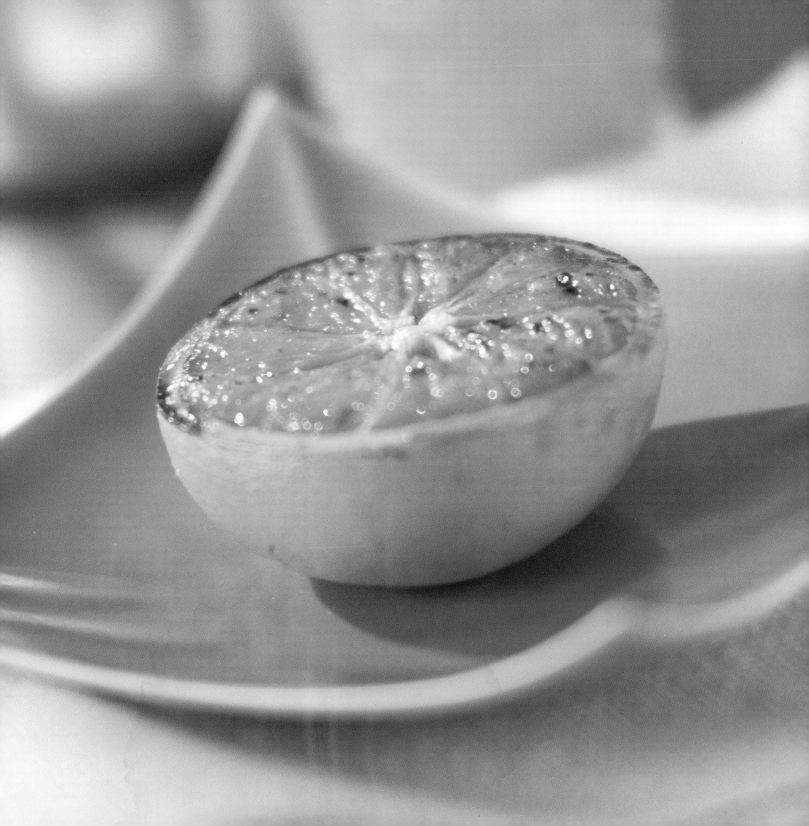

broiled scallop *and* oyster brochettes

These delicious seafood brochettes are an ideal summertime dish, perfect for barbecues. Seafood and shellfish contain zinc and also tyrosine, an amino acid used to make brain-stimulating chemicals that increase mental alertness.

ingredients

- 16 medium or large shucked raw scallops
- 16 shucked raw oysters
- 16 shucked raw shrimp (or king shrimp)
- 2 small yellow bell peppers, seeded and cut into 8 pieces
- 1 zucchini, cut into 16 thin slices
- 16 small ready-to-eat dried apricots
- 4tbsp olive oil
- 2tbsp unsweetened apple juice
- 1 clove garlic, crushed
- 2tbsp chopped fresh mixed herbs
- sea salt
- freshly ground black pepper

serves *four*
preparation time *10 minutes, plus 1 hour marinating time*
cooking time *8–10 minutes*

method

1 Thread the scallops, oysters, shrimps, vegetables, and apricots onto four long skewers, dividing the ingredients evenly among them. Place the skewers in a shallow, nonmetallic dish.
2 Put the oil, apple juice, garlic, herbs, and seasoning in a small bowl and whisk until thoroughly mixed. Drizzle over the brochettes; then turn the brochettes over in the marinade to coat them completely. Cover and leave to marinate in the refrigerator for 1 hour.
3 Preheat the broiler to high. Place the brochettes on a rack in a broiler pan and broil for 8–10 minutes, until cooked, turning occasionally. Brush frequently with the marinade during cooking, to prevent the brochettes drying out.
4 Serve the hot brochettes with cooked fresh vegetables such as new potatoes, zucchini, and corn.

variations

- *Use mushrooms instead of apricots.*
- *Use unsweetened orange juice or white grape juice instead of apple.*
- *Use chopped fresh flat-leaf parsley instead of mixed herbs.*

fish *dishes*

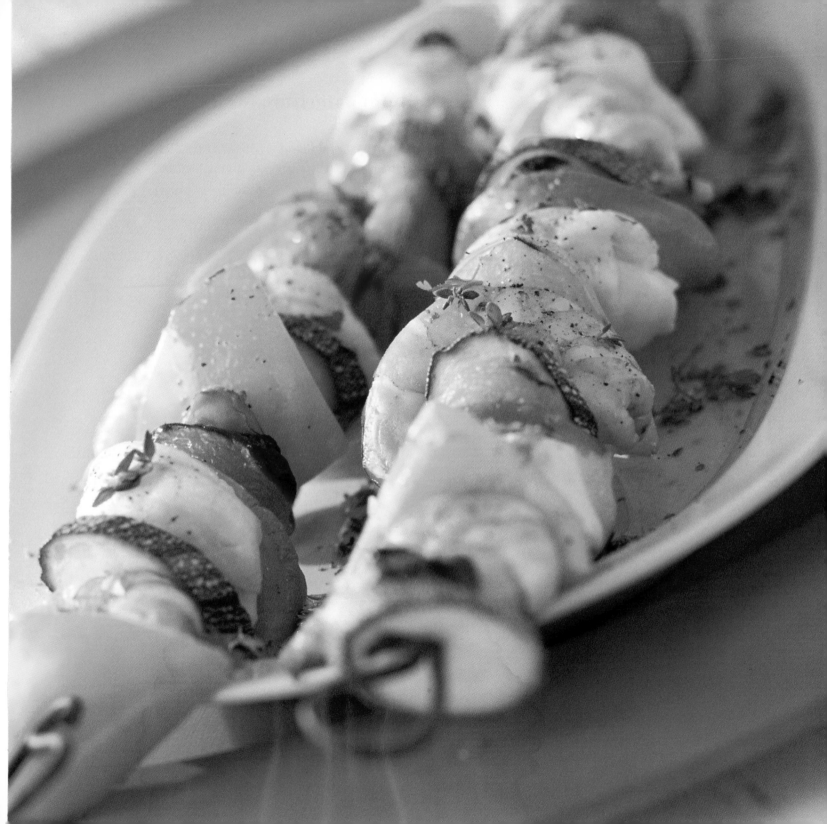

chicken breasts stuffed *with* mushrooms *and* sage

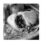 This tasty way of serving chicken is sure to be popular with the whole family. Fresh sage is considered to be a mild stimulant.

▌ ingredients

- 1 tbsp/½ ounce (15g) butter
- 4 shallots (French shallots), finely chopped
- 1 clove garlic, crushed
- 1 small leek, finely chopped
- 1⅓ cups/4 ounces (115g) cremini mushrooms, finely chopped
- 1 tbsp chopped fresh sage
- 1 tsp finely grated lemon rind
- sea salt
- freshly ground black pepper
- 4 large skinless, boneless chicken breasts
- 2 tbsp olive oil
- fresh sage leaves, to garnish

serves *four*
preparation time *30 minutes*
cooking time *30–45 minutes*

▌ method

1 Preheat the oven to 400°F.
2 Lightly grease a baking tray.
3 Melt the butter in a saucepan. Add the shallots, garlic, leek, and mushrooms, and cook gently for about 10 minutes, stirring occasionally, until softened.
4 Remove the pan from the heat. Stir in the chopped sage, lemon rind, and seasoning.
5 Place the chicken breasts on a flat surface. Cover loosely with a sheet of baking parchment and pound with a rolling pin to an even thickness. Remove and discard the baking parchment.
6 Spoon some mushroom mixture across the center of each breast; then fold one end over the filling and overlap the other end over the top to make a package. Secure with toothpicks. Brush the chicken all over with oil and place, seam-side down, on the prepared baking tray.
7 Bake for 30–45 minutes, until the chicken is cooked through and tender. Remove the toothpicks before serving.

8 Garnish with fresh sage leaves and serve hot with brown rice and cooked fresh vegetables such as spinach and rutabaga.

variations
- *Use turkey instead of chicken.*
- *Use fresh thyme instead of sage.*
- *Use fresh wild (field) mushrooms instead of cremini mushrooms.*

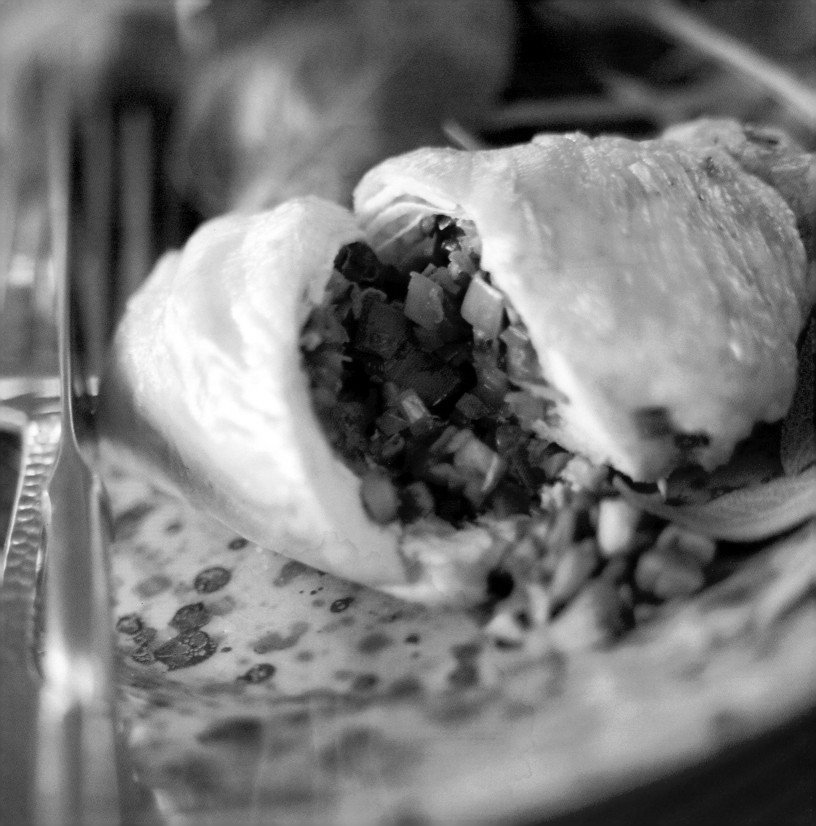

vegetable *and* parsley bake

 This potato-topped vegetable bake makes a good family dish. Parsley is a source of iron and vitamin C, which helps the absorption of iron.

■ ingredients

- 6 cups/2 pounds (900g) diced potatoes
- 2tbsp of butter
- 2tbsp chopped fresh chives
- 2 cups/16 fluid ounces (450ml) plus 2 tbsp milk
- sea salt
- freshly ground black pepper
- 2 leeks, washed and sliced
- 6 ounces (175g) mushrooms, sliced
- 2 cups/12 ounces (350g) frozen peas
- 3 tbsp/1½ ounces (40g) butter
- 5 tbsp/1½ ounces (40g) whole-wheat flour
- ½tsp mustard
- ¾ cup/3 ounces (85g) grated Cheddar cheese
- 1 7-ounce (200g) can corn kernels, drained
- 3–4tbsp chopped fresh parsley
- fresh parsley sprigs, to garnish

serves *four to six*
preparation time *30 minutes*
cooking time *25–30 minutes*

■ method

1 Preheat the oven to 375°F.
2 Boil the potatoes for 10–15 minutes, until tender. Drain and mash. Stir in the 2tbsp of butter, chives, 2tbsp of the milk, and seasoning.
3 Steam the leeks and mushrooms over a saucepan of boiling water for 10 minutes. Add the peas and steam for another 3–5 minutes, until tender.
4 Put the remaining milk, 3 tbsp/1½ ounces (40g) butter, the flour, and mustard in a saucepan. Heat gently, whisking continuously, until the sauce comes to a boil and thickens. Simmer gently for 2 minutes, stirring.
5 Remove the pan from the heat and stir in the cheese, leeks, mushrooms, peas, corn, parsley, and seasoning.
6 Spoon into an ovenproof dish and spoon the mashed potato over the top, covering the mixture.
7 Bake for 25–30 minutes, until the potato is crisp.
8 Garnish with parsley sprigs and serve with cooked vegetables.

honey-glazed baby carrots

These delicious, honey-glazed carrots are an ideal accompaniment to broiled lean meat or fish. Vegetarians will enjoy them with a mixed vegetable pilaf or potato bake. Carrots contain B vitamins.

■ ingredients

- 1 pound (450g) baby (Dutch) carrots
- 2 tbsp/1 ounce (25g) butter
- 3tbsp honey
- 2tsp chopped fresh thyme
- sea salt
- freshly ground black pepper
- fresh thyme sprigs, to garnish

serves *four as an accompaniment*
preparation time *10 minutes*
cooking time *15–20 minutes*

■ method

1 Cook the carrots in a saucepan of boiling water for 3 minutes. Drain well and set aside.
2 Put the butter and honey in a saucepan and heat gently until melted. Add the carrots, chopped thyme, and seasoning, and mix well. Cover and cook gently for 10–15 minutes, until the carrots are tender and glazed all over, stirring occasionally.
3 Garnish with the thyme sprigs and serve hot with broiled lean meat or fish and boiled new potatoes with mint.

variations

- *Use maple syrup instead of honey.*
- *Use baby corn instead of carrots.*

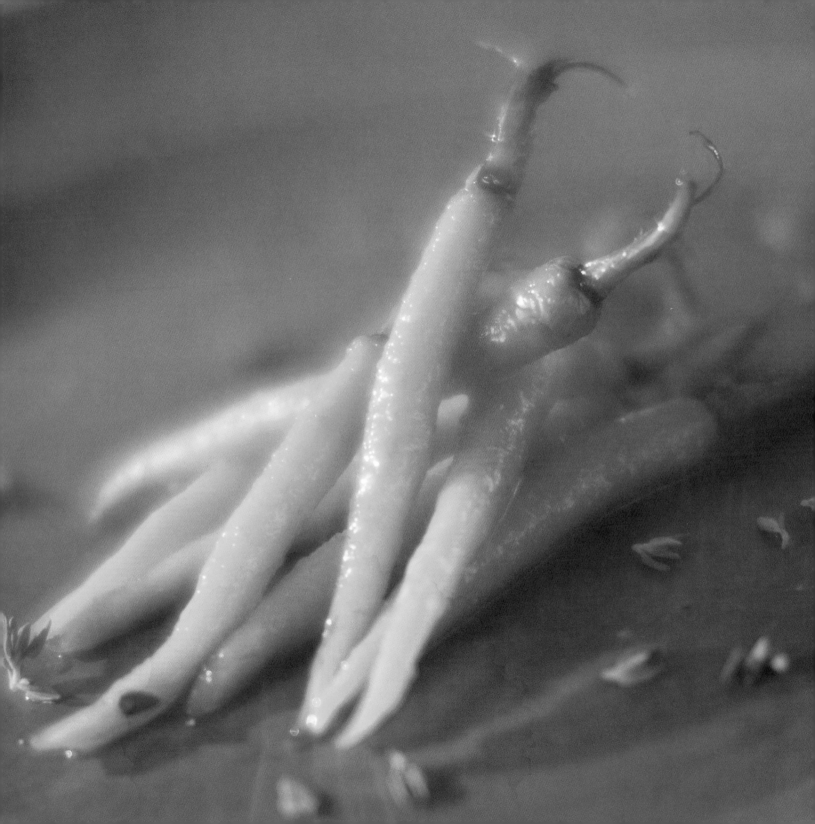

broccoli *and* zucchini millet pilaf

Millet pilaf makes a change from rice pilaf and is ideal for a family meal. Millet is a good source of B group vitamins, which are important for healthy brain function. Broccoli contains vitamin C and beta carotene.

■ ingredients

- 1 tbsp olive oil
- 3½ cups/12 ounces (350g) chopped shallots (French shallots),
- 1 red bell pepper, seeded and diced
- 1 clove garlic, crushed
- 2 zucchini, sliced
- 1¼ cups/8 ounces (225g) millet seed
- 2 cups/16 fluid ounces (450ml) vegetable stock (see recipe on page 20)
- ⅔ cup/¼ pint (150ml) dry white wine
- ⅔ cup/4 ounces (115g) golden raisins
- 1 tsp ground cinnamon
- sea salt
- freshly ground black pepper
- 10 ounces (280g) small broccoli florets
- 1–2 tbsp chopped fresh mixed herbs
- fresh herb sprigs, to garnish

serves *four to six*
preparation time *10 minutes*
cooking time *20–25 minutes*

■ method

1 Heat the oil in a large saucepan. Add the shallots, red bell pepper, and garlic, and cook for 5 minutes, stirring occasionally.
2 Add the zucchini, millet, stock, wine, golden raisins, cinnamon, and seasoning, and mix well. Cover and bring to a boil; then reduce the heat and simmer for 15–20 minutes, until all the liquid has been absorbed and the millet is tender, stirring occasionally.
3 Meanwhile, cook the broccoli in boiling water for about 5 minutes, until cooked and tender. Drain well and keep warm.
4 Fold the broccoli and herbs into the pilaf. Garnish with the herb sprigs and serve hot with a mixed tomato and bell pepper salad.

variations

- *Use onions instead of shallots.*
- *Use sliced mushrooms or corn kernels instead of golden raisins.*
- *Use chopped ready-to-eat dried apricots instead of golden raisins.*

freezing instructions

Let cool completely, then transfer to a rigid, freezeproof container. Cover, seal, and label. Freeze for up to 3 months. Defrost for several hours, or overnight in the refrigerator. Reheat gently in a saucepan until piping hot, adding a little extra stock if necessary.

vegetable *dishes*

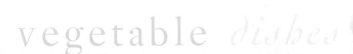

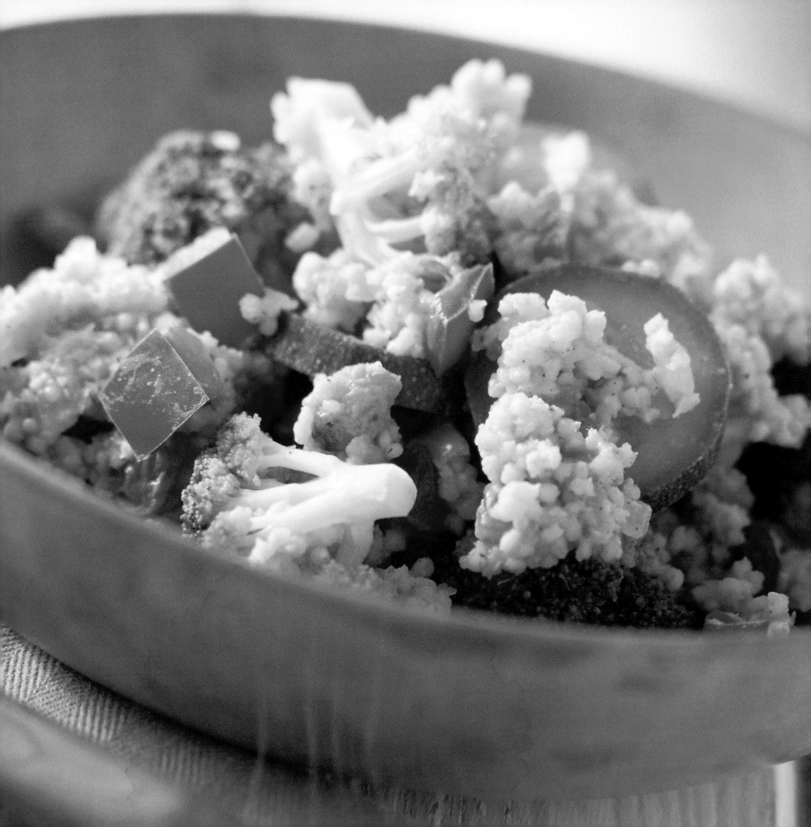

fresh figs *with* vanilla yogurt

Enjoy fresh figs when they are at their best, served with vanilla yogurt. Fresh figs provide small amounts of the many vitamins and minerals necessary for a healthy brain and nervous system.

ingredients

- ¾ cup/7 ounces (200g) plain yogurt
- 1–2tbsp honey
- a few drops of vanilla extract
- 8 fresh figs
- finely grated dark chocolate, for sprinkling (optional)

serves *four*
preparation time *15 minutes*

method

1 Put the yogurt, honey, and vanilla extract in a bowl and gently fold together. Cover and chill in the refrigerator while preparing the figs.

2 Using a sharp knife, cut the stalk ends off the figs; then cut a deep cross in the top of each fruit. Using your fingers, gently press each fig open to make four "petals."

3 Spoon some vanilla yogurt into the center of each fig, or alongside the fruit, and serve immediately, sprinkled with a little grated chocolate, if liked.

variations

- *Use almond extract instead of vanilla extract.*
- *Use maple syrup instead of honey.*
- *Serve the vanilla yogurt with other prepared fresh fruit, such as passionfruit, nectarines, or peaches.*

cherry batter dessert

This fruity, oven-baked batter dessert will be popular with all the family. Cherries contain vitamin C, which the body needs in greater amounts when under stress.

ingredients

- 1 cup/4 ounces (115g) whole-wheat flour
- ½ cup/2 ounces (55g) sugar
- 1tsp ground cinnamon
- 1 medium egg
- 1¼ cups/½ pint (300ml) milk
- 12 ounces (350g) pitted, fresh or canned (drained), sweet black cherries
- 1tbsp sunflower oil

serves *four*
preparation time *15 minutes*
cooking time *25–30 minutes*

method

1 Preheat the oven to 425°F.

2 Put the flour, sugar, and cinnamon in a bowl and stir; then make a well in the center. Break in the egg and add a little milk, beating well with a wooden spoon. Gradually beat in the remaining milk, drawing the flour mixture in from the sides, to make a smooth batter.

3 Put the oil in a 7-by-11-inch baking pan (18x28cm) and put in the oven for 2–3 minutes, until hot. Quickly scatter the cherries over the bottom; then pour the batter evenly over the fruit. Bake for 25–30 minutes, until risen and golden brown.

4 Cut the cherry batter dessert into squares and serve hot or cold, with a little plain yogurt.

variations

- *Use half whole-wheat and half buckwheat flour instead of all whole-wheat flour.*
- *Use ginger instead of cinnamon.*

desserts *and* bakes

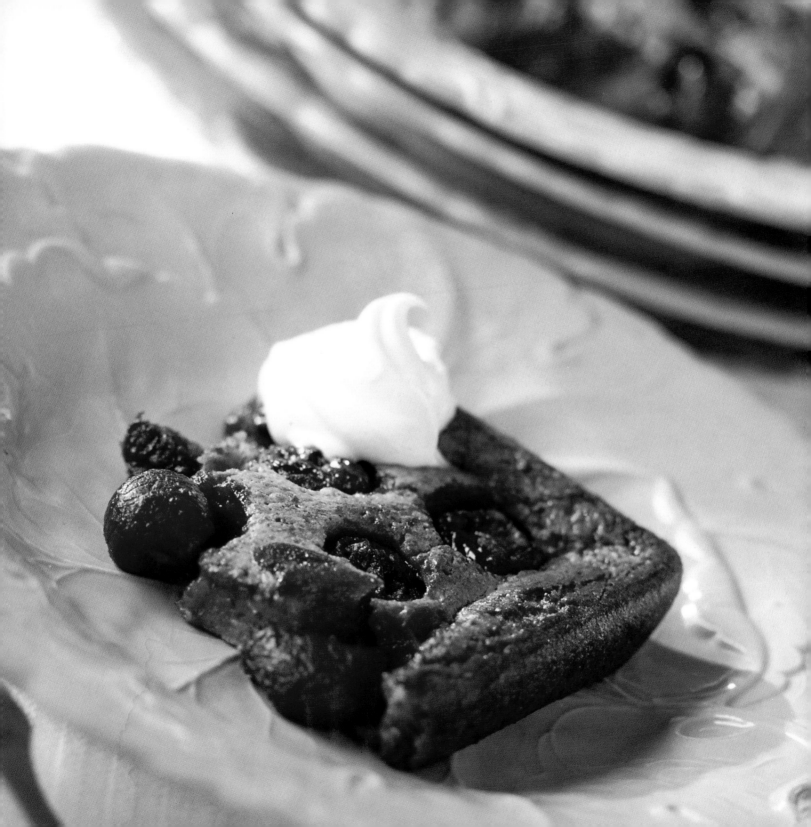

iced terrine of summer fruits

 This creamy, iced terrine is an ideal warm weather dessert to enjoy alfresco. Yogurt is a good source of protein, calcium, and B vitamins.

ingredients

- 1 pound (450g) ripe mixed summer fruits, such as strawberries, raspberries, blueberries, blackberries, cherries, and redcurrants
- ½ cup/2 ounces (55g) light brown sugar
- scant 1¼ cups/10 ounces (280g) raspberry yogurt
- ⅔ cup/¼ pint (150ml) light cream
- ⅔ cup/5 ounces (140g) crème fraîche or light sour cream
- fresh mint sprigs, to decorate

serves *six to eight*
preparation time *20 minutes, plus freezing time*

method

1 Line a 2-pound (900g) loaf pan with plastic freezer wrap and set aside.
2 Put the mixed fruits in a food processor and blend until smooth. Press the purée through a sieve, discarding the seeds and reserving the juice and pulp.
3 Return the fruit pulp and juices to the rinsed-out food processor bowl. Add the sugar, yogurt, cream, and crème fraîche or light sour cream, and blend until well mixed.
4 Pour the mixture into a chilled, shallow, plastic container. Cover and freeze for 1½–2 hours, or until the mixture has a mushy consistency. Spoon into a bowl and mash with a fork to break down the ice crystals.

5 Pour the mixture into the prepared loaf pan and level the surface. Freeze until firm.
6 Turn the terrine out onto a serving plate and peel off and discard the plastic wrap. Place in the refrigerator for 30 minutes before serving, to soften a little.
7 Decorate with the mint sprigs and serve in slices with fresh fruit, such as apricots and peaches.

variations
- *Use other mixtures of fruits.*
- *Use the same quantity of frozen fruits (defrosted), instead of fresh.*

freezing instructions
This iced terrine will keep for up to 3 months in the freezer.

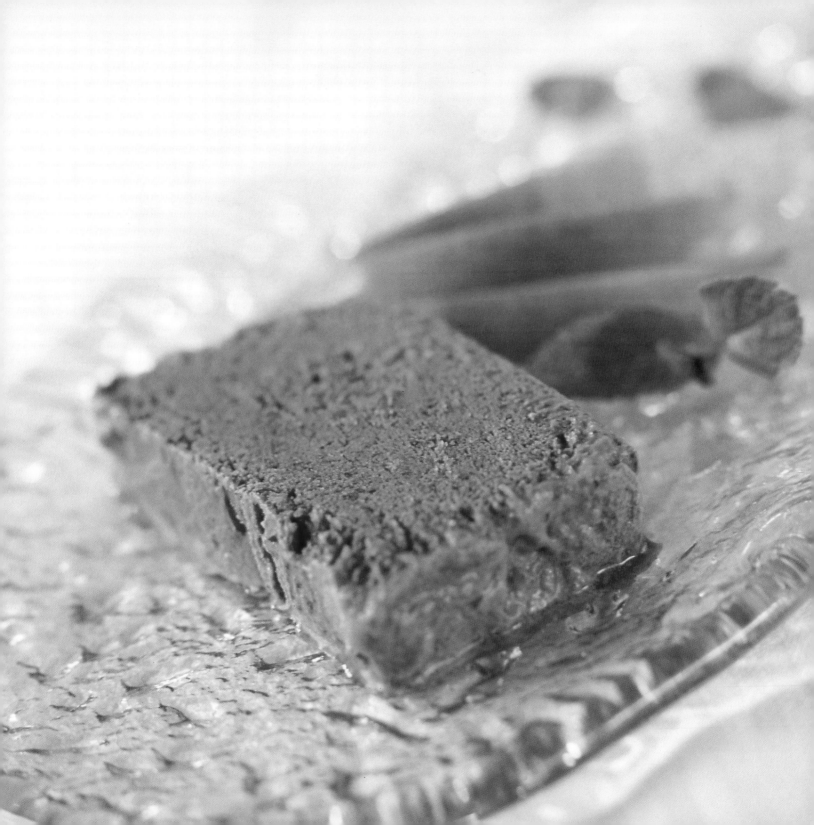

celebration banquet

EPRESSED AND WORN *out? Dine your way to tranquility and happiness—this selection of recipes from the feel-good foods* section *is an ideal antidote to a stressful day, full of reviving nutrients such as protein and vitamin C. So dig in to lift your mood!*

pink grapefruit *with* cinnamon

Start off this de-stressing menu with a sweet, vitamin C-rich grapefruit.

■ ingredients

- 2 pink grapefruit
- 2tbsp light brown sugar
- 1–2tsp ground cinnamon
- fresh mint sprigs, to garnish (optional)

serves *four*
preparation time *10 minutes*
cooking time *3–5 minutes*

■ method

1 Preheat the broiler to medium. Cut each grapefruit in half; then cut between the segments to loosen the flesh.
2 Mix the sugar and cinnamon together and sprinkle over the grapefruit.
3 Place the grapefruit on a broiler rack in a broiler pan and broil for a few minutes, until the sugar has melted and the grapefruit are hot.
4 Serve immediately, garnished with the mint sprigs, if liked.

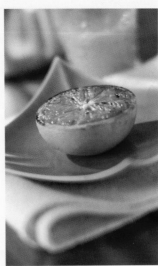

chicken breasts stuffed *with* mushrooms and sage

These chicken breasts are pepped up with sprigs of stimulating sage.

■ ingredients

- 1 tbsp/½ ounce (15g) butter
- 4 shallots (French shallots), finely chopped
- 1 clove garlic, crushed
- 1 small leek, finely chopped
- 1⅓ cups/4 ounces (115g) cremini mushrooms, finely chopped
- 1tbsp chopped fresh sage
- 1tsp finely grated lemon rind
- sea salt
- freshly ground black pepper
- 4 large skinless, boneless chicken breasts
- 2tbsp olive oil
- fresh sage leaves, to garnish

serves *four*
preparation time *30 minutes*
cooking time *30–45 minutes*

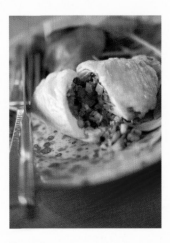

method

1 Preheat the oven to 400°F.

2 Lightly grease a baking tray.

3 Melt the butter in a saucepan. Add the shallots, garlic, leek, and mushrooms, and cook gently for about 10 minutes, stirring occasionally, until softened.

4 Remove the pan from the heat. Stir in the chopped sage, lemon rind, and seasoning.

5 Place the chicken breasts on a flat surface. Cover loosely with a sheet of baking parchment and pound with a rolling pin to an even thickness. Remove and discard the baking parchment.

6 Spoon some mushroom mixture across the center of each breast; then fold one end over the filling and overlap the other end over the top to make a package. Secure with toothpicks. Brush the chicken all over with oil and place, seam-side down, on the prepared baking tray.

7 Bake for 30–45 minutes, until the chicken is cooked through and tender. Remove the toothpicks before serving.

8 Garnish with fresh sage leaves and serve hot with brown rice and cooked fresh vegetables such as spinach and rutabaga.

iced terrine of summer fruits

Yogurt makes for a protein-rich, soothing, and nutritious dessert.

ingredients

- 1 pound (450g) ripe mixed summer fruits, such as strawberries, raspberries, blueberries, blackberries, cherries, and redcurrants
- ½ cup/2 ounces (55g) light brown sugar
- scant 1¼ cups/10 ounces (280g) raspberry yogurt
- ⅔ cup/¼ pint (150ml) light cream
- ⅔ cup/5 ounces (140g) crème fraîche or light sour cream
- fresh mint sprigs, to decorate

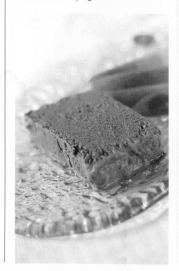

serves *six to eight*
preparation time *20 minutes, plus freezing time*

method

1 Line a 2-pound (900g) loaf pan with plastic freezer wrap and set aside.

2 Put the mixed fruits in a food processor and blend until smooth. Press the purée through a sieve, discarding the seeds and reserving the juice and pulp.

3 Return the fruit pulp and juices to the rinsed-out food processor bowl. Add the sugar, yogurt, cream, and crème fraîche or light sour cream, and blend until well mixed.

4 Pour the mixture into a chilled, shallow, plastic container. Cover and freeze for 1½–2 hours, or until the mixture has a mushy consistency. Spoon into a bowl and mash with a fork to break down the ice crystals.

5 Pour the mixture into the prepared loaf pan and level the surface. Freeze until firm.

6 Turn the terrine out onto a serving plate and peel off and discard the plastic wrap. Place in the refrigerator for 30 minutes before serving, to soften a little.

7 Decorate with the mint sprigs and serve in slices with fresh fruit, such as apricots and peaches.

reviving *foods*

A DEFICIENCY IN MINERALS *can have a profound effect on mood. A lack of calcium and magnesium can cause depression, tenseness, and irritability. No one should be short of either of these minerals if they eat plenty of fresh and dried fruit, green and root vegetables, fish, low-fat dairy products such as yogurt and cheese, legumes, nuts, and seafood. Some areas of the brain have high concentrations of iron, and it is thought that a lowering of iron levels could also trigger mood changes. Foods that are rich in iron are lean meats, dark-meat poultry, shellfish, fish, green leafy vegetables, dried fruit, nuts, and enriched grains.*

green bean vinaigrette

This quick and easy dish makes a good appetizer or side dish. Green beans contain iron, calcium, magnesium, boron, vitamin C, and B vitamins, important nutrients for a healthy nervous system and brain function.

▌ ingredients

- 1½ pounds (700g) string beans, trimmed
- ⅔ cup/¼ pint (150ml) French dressing (see recipe on page 21)
- ½ cup/2 ounces (55g) toasted flaked almonds

serves *six*
preparation time *10 minutes*
cooking time *5–6 minutes*

▌ method

1 Cook the beans in a large saucepan of lightly salted, boiling water for 5–6 minutes, until tender but still crisp. Drain well.
2 Serve the beans hot or cold, with the French dressing drizzled over the top. Sprinkle with flaked almonds just before serving.
3 Serve with crusty whole-wheat bread or bread rolls.

variations

- *Use baby (Dutch) carrots or baby corn instead of beans.*
- *Use chopped toasted hazelnuts instead of almonds.*
- *Serve the beans as an accompaniment to broiled lean meat or fish with baked potatoes.*

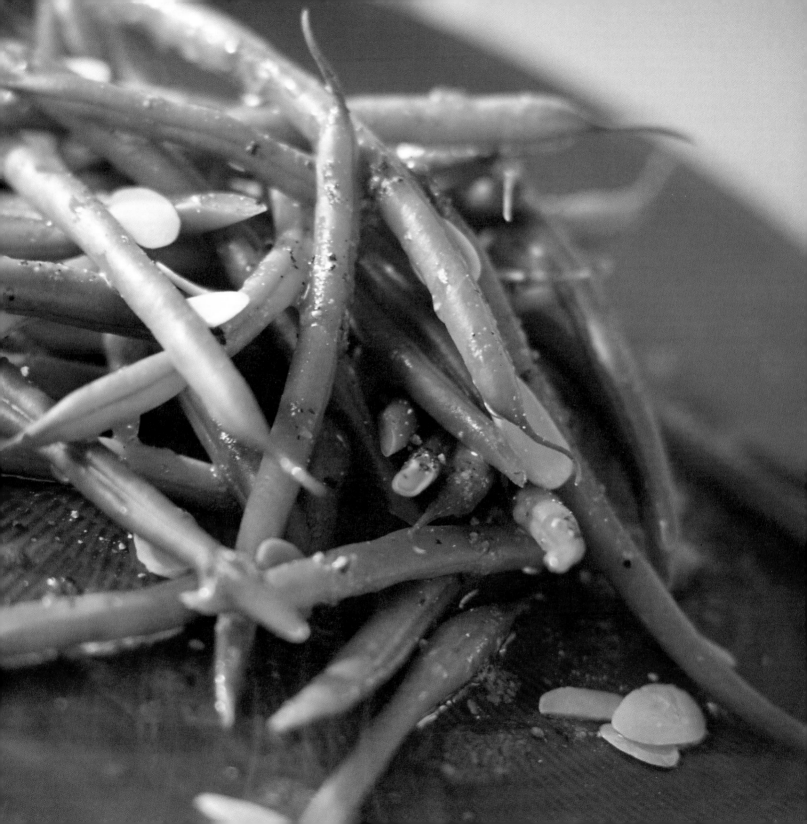

turkey waldorf salad

The addition of turkey increases the flavor and nutrients of this tasty salad. Walnuts contain essential fatty acids that are especially important for healthy brain tissue and an efficient nervous system.

■ ingredients

- 6tbsp mayonnaise (see recipe on page 21)
- 4tbsp plain yogurt
- 2 red-skinned eating apples
- 1tbsp fresh lemon juice
- 1¾ cups/8 ounces (225g) diced, cold, cooked, skinless, boneless turkey breast
- 4 celery stalks, chopped
- ½ cup/2 ounces (55g) roughly chopped walnuts
- 2tbsp chopped fresh chives
- sea salt
- freshly ground black pepper
- 1 round (butterhead) lettuce, shredded
- fresh chive flowers, to garnish

serves *four*
preparation time *15 minutes*

■ method

1 Mix the mayonnaise and yogurt in a small bowl and set aside.
2 Core and dice the apples and toss them in the lemon juice.
3 Put the apples in a bowl with the turkey, celery, walnuts, and chopped chives, and stir.
4 Add the mayonnaise mixture and toss to mix well. Season to taste with salt and pepper.
5 Arrange the lettuce leaves on a serving plate or platter and spoon the salad on top. Garnish with fresh chive flowers and serve immediately with slices of whole-wheat bread.

variations

• *Use mushrooms instead of turkey.*
• *Use pears instead of apples.*
• *Use pecans or cashews instead of walnuts.*
• *Use cooked chicken breast instead of turkey.*

noodle salad *with* sesame seeds

This warm noodle salad can be served as a filling appetizer or a snack. Sesame seeds contain iron, magnesium, and calcium, all important nutrients for a healthy nervous system.

■ ingredients

- 4tbsp unsweetened orange juice
- 1tbsp olive oil
- 1tbsp light soy sauce
- 1tbsp red wine vinegar
- 1tbsp honey
- 1tbsp tomato purée (paste)
- 1tbsp dry sherry
- 1 clove garlic, crushed
- sea salt and ground black pepper
- 8 ounces (250g) cherry tomatoes, halved
- ¾ cup/3 ounces (85g) chopped sugar-snap peas (mangetout)
- ½ cup/3 ounces (85g) sliced radishes
- 1 yellow bell pepper, seeded and diced
- 4 green onions, chopped
- 1 14-ounce (400g) can green beans, rinsed and drained
- 6 ounces (175g) dried egg noodles, broken into short lengths
- 2–3tbsp toasted sesame seeds
- fresh herb sprigs, to garnish

serves *six*
preparation time *15 minutes*
cooking time *4 minutes*

■ method

1 Put the orange juice, oil, soy sauce, vinegar, honey, tomato paste, sherry, garlic, and seasoning in a small bowl and whisk.
2 Put the tomatoes, sugar-snap peas, radishes, yellow pepper, green onions, and green beans in a bowl and stir.
3 Cook the noodles in boiling water for about 4 minutes, or according to the package directions. Drain well.
4 Give the dressing a quick whisk; then pour it over the hot noodles and toss.
5 Add the noodles to the vegetables and toss together.
6 Sprinkle with sesame seeds and garnish with fresh herb sprigs. Serve with whole-wheat rolls.

variations

• *Use baby corn, bean sprouts, and Chinese cabbage (greens) instead of cherry tomatoes, sugar-snap peas, and radishes.*
• *Use unsweetened white grape juice or apple juice instead of orange juice.*
• *Use canned kidney beans or black-eyed peas instead of green beans.*

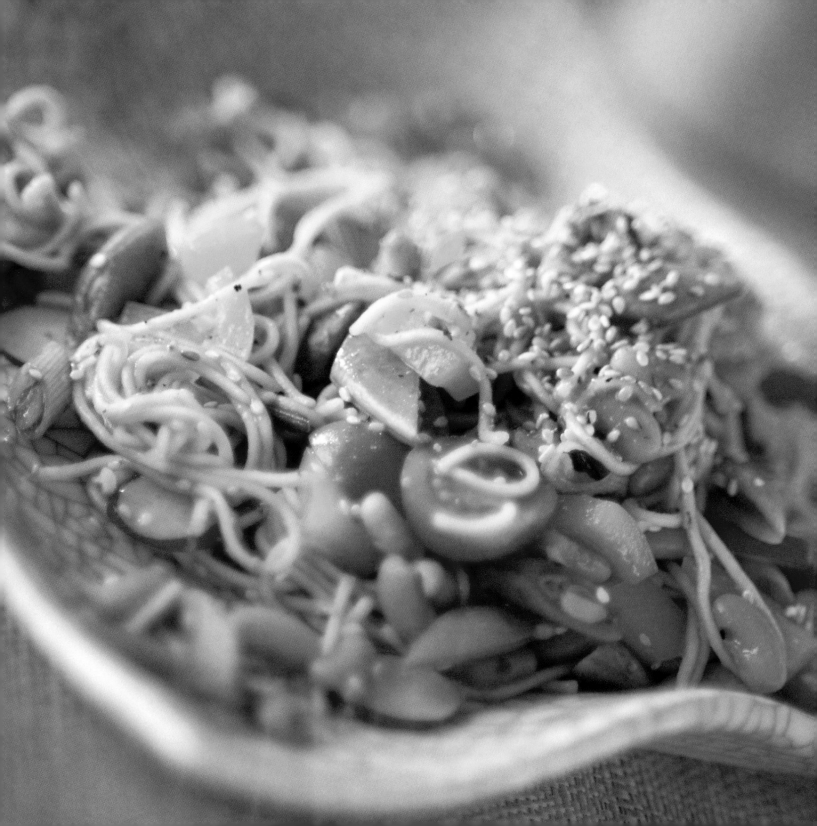

tuna steaks *with* mussel *and* white wine sauce

Succulent tuna steaks oven-baked and served with a white wine and mussel sauce make a flavorsome dish. Fresh fish is a good source of protein, B vitamins, and minerals that are important for healthy brain and nerve function.

■ ingredients

- 4 tuna steaks, each weighing about 6 ounces (175g)
- juice of 2 limes
- fresh flat-leaf parsley sprigs, to garnish

for the sauce

- 2 tbsp cornstarch
- 1½ cups/12 fluid ounces (350ml) dry or medium-dry white wine
- 7 ounces (200g) cooked, shucked mussels (halved, if preferred)
- 1 tbsp/½ ounce (15g) butter
- 3 tbsp crème fraîche or light sour cream
- 2 tbsp chopped, fresh flatleaf parsley
- sea salt
- freshly ground black pepper

serves *four*
preparation time *10 minutes*
cooking time *20–25 minutes*

■ method

1 Preheat the oven to 350°F.
2 Cut four pieces of nonstick baking parchment, each large enough to wrap one tuna steak. Place a tuna steak on each and drizzle over some lime juice. Fold the parchment over the fish and twist the edges to secure.
3 Place the packages on a baking tray and bake for 20–25 minutes, until the fish is cooked and the flesh just flakes when tested with a fork.
4 Meanwhile, make the sauce. In a saucepan, blend the cornstarch with a little of the wine. Stir in the remaining wine; then heat gently, stirring constantly, until the sauce comes to a boil and thickens. Simmer gently for 2 minutes, stirring.
5 Stir in the mussels, butter, crème fraîche, parsley, and seasoning, and heat gently until piping hot.

6 Open the package carefully and place the steaks on warmed serving plates. Pour some sauce over each one.
7 Garnish with parsley sprigs and serve with new potatoes, carrots and celery.

variations

- *Use salmon steaks instead of tuna.*
- *Use lemon juice instead of lime.*
- *Use cooked, shelled shrimp instead of mussels.*
- *Use red wine instead of white wine.*

fish *dishes*

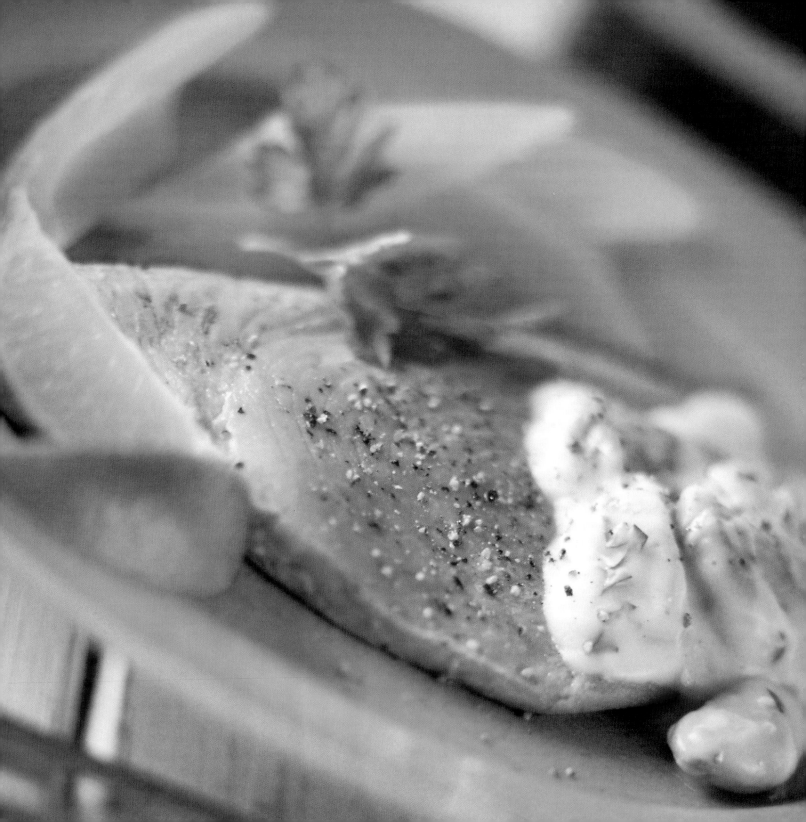

seafood paella

This delicious seafood paella makes a nutritious and substantial meal. Seafood is a good source of protein, B vitamins, and minerals that support normal brain function.

ingredients

- 1tbsp olive oil
- 1 onion, chopped
- 2 cloves garlic, finely chopped
- 1 red bell pepper, seeded and diced
- 1¼ cups/8 ounces (225g) long-grain brown rice
- 8 ounces (225g) raw, shelled tiger (or king) shrimp, plus 4 cooked shrimp in their shells, to garnish
- 8 ounces (225g) prepared raw squid, sliced into rings
- large dash of saffron threads, crushed
- 1¼ cups/½ pint (300ml) vegetable stock (see recipe on page 20)
- 1¼ cups/½ pint (300ml) dry white wine
- ⅔ cup/4 ounces (115g) fresh or frozen peas
- 3 tomatoes, peeled and chopped
- sea salt
- freshly ground black pepper
- 8 ounces (225g) fresh raw mussels in their shells, scrubbed and debearded
- 2tbsp chopped fresh parsley

serves *four*
preparation time *15 minutes*
cooking time *45 minutes*

method

1 Heat the oil in a large nonstick skillet or paella pan. Add the onion, garlic, and red bell pepper, and cook gently for 5 minutes, stirring occasionally.

2 Add the rice, shrimp, and squid, and cook gently for 5 minutes, stirring occasionally.

3 Stir in the saffron threads, stock, wine, peas, tomatoes, and seasoning. Bring to a boil, stirring constantly. Reduce the heat and simmer, uncovered, for about 35 minutes, until most of the stock has been absorbed and the rice is cooked, stirring occasionally.

4 Meanwhile, cook the mussels in a saucepan of boiling water for about 5 minutes, until the shells open. Drain, and discard any mussels that remain closed.

5 Stir the mussels and parsley into the paella and serve immediately, garnished with whole shrimp and lemon wedges.

6 Serve with whole-wheat bread or a mixed leaf and carrot salad.

variations

- *Use fresh raw scallops instead of the shrimp or the squid.*
- *Use mushrooms instead of peas.*
- *Use 2 leeks instead of the onion.*

fish *dishes*

stir-fried chicken livers *with* mixed greens

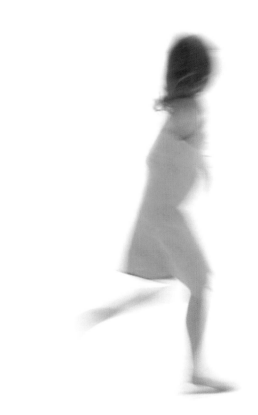

When eaten occasionally, tender chicken livers make a nutritious dish. Liver is a good source of B vitamins and iron, both of which are good for normal brain function.

■ ingredients

- 1 tbsp cornstarch
- 6 tbsp medium-dry cider
- 2 tbsp light soy sauce
- 1 tbsp whole-grain mustard
- sea salt
- freshly ground black pepper
- 1–2 tbsp olive oil
- 12 ounces (350g) chicken livers, cut into thin strips
- 2 leeks, washed and thinly sliced
- 1 red bell pepper, seeded and sliced
- 1 yellow bell pepper, seeded and sliced
- 2 cups/4 ounces (115g) shredded spinach
- 1½ cup/3 ounces (85g) shredded green (crinkle-leafed) cabbage,
- fresh herb sprigs, to garnish

serves *four*
preparation time *15 minutes*
cooking time *5–7 minutes*

■ method

1 In a small bowl, blend the cornstarch with the cider; then add the soy sauce, mustard, and seasoning. Set aside.

2 Heat the oil in a wok or large skillet. Add the liver and stir-fry over a high heat for 1 minute.

3 Add the leeks, peppers, spinach, and cabbage. Stir-fry for 3–4 minutes.

4 Add the reserved cornstarch mixture. Stir-fry for 1–2 minutes until the sauce is thickened and glossy and the liver and vegetables are cooked and tender.

5 Garnish with the herb sprigs and serve with mashed potatoes, carrots, and green beans.

variations

- *Use 1 onion instead of the leeks.*
- *Use 1 zucchini instead of the yellow pepper.*
- *Use Chinese cabbage (greens) instead of cabbage.*

meat *and* poultry *dishes*

shredded duck *with* ginger *and* lime

Duck breast marinated in lime and ginger and stir-fried with vegetables makes a delicious, warming meal. Some say ginger is an aid to digestion and helps to lift the mood. Limes are an excellent source of vitamin C.

ingredients

- finely grated zest and juice of 1 lime
- 1 tsp ground ginger
- 1 tbsp dry sherry
- 1 tbsp light soy sauce
- sea salt
- freshly ground black pepper
- 12 ounces (350g) skinless, boneless duck breast, cut into thin strips
- 1 tbsp olive oil
- 1 small red chili, seeded and finely chopped
- 1 clove garlic, crushed
- 1-inch (2.5cm) piece fresh ginger root, peeled and finely chopped
- 1 yellow bell pepper, seeded and sliced
- 6–8 green onions, chopped
- 6 ounces (175g) baby corn
- 4 ounces (115g) sugar-snap peas (mangetout)
- toasted sesame seeds, to garnish

serves *four*
preparation time *15 minutes, plus 20 minutes marinating time*
cooking time *8–10 minutes*

method

1 Put the lime zest and juice, ground ginger, sherry, soy sauce, and seasoning in a bowl and whisk. Add the duck and toss to mix well. Cover and refrigerate for 20 minutes.

2 Using a slotted spoon, remove the duck from the marinade, and reserve the marinade.

3 Heat the oil in a nonstick wok or large skillet. Add the chili, garlic, and ginger root, and stir-fry over a high heat for 30 seconds.

4 Add the duck and stir-fry for 1–2 minutes until lightly browned.

5 Add the yellow pepper, green onions, corn, and sugar-snap peas and stir-fry for another 3–4 minutes.

6 Add the marinade and stir-fry for 2–3 minutes, until the duck is cooked through.

7 Sprinkle with sesame seeds and serve with egg or rice noodles and a mixed dark-green leaf salad.

variations

- *Use sliced fresh wild (field) mushrooms instead of sugar-snap peas.*
- *Use lean chicken, turkey, or lamb instead of duck.*
- *Use 1 lemon instead of lime.*

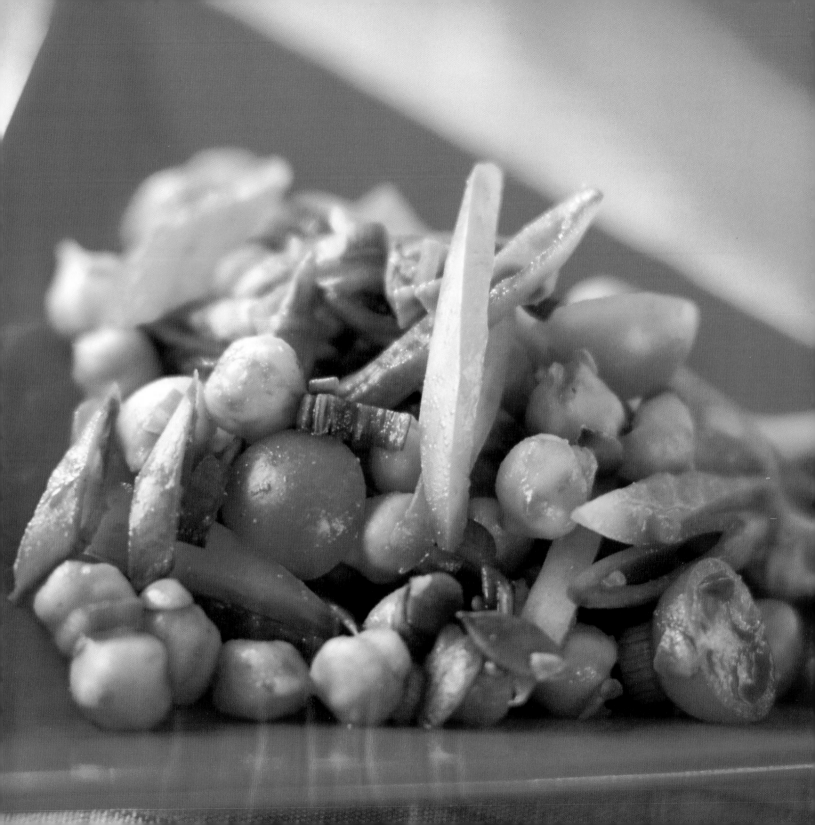

fruit *and* nut chocolate slices

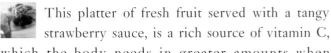

These chocolate slices are hard to resist for a special treat. Dried fruit and nuts contain many nutrients including B vitamins, boron, iron, and magnesium, all vital nutrients for healthy brain function.

■ ingredients

- 6 squares/6 ounces (175g) dark chocolate, broken into pieces
- ½ cup/4 ounces (115g) butter
- 1 tbsp maple syrup
- 2 tbsp brandy
- 1½ cups/6 ounces (175g) mixed dried fruit, including golden raisins and chopped ready-to-eat dried pineapple, dates, peaches, and pears
- ½ cup/2 ounces (55g) roughly chopped Brazil nuts
- ½ cup/2 ounces (55g) halved cashews

makes 24 *small bars or squares*
preparation time *15 minutes, plus chilling time*

■ method

1 Lightly grease and line an 8-inch (20cm) square cake pan.
2 Put the chocolate, butter, and syrup in a medium-size bowl over a saucepan of simmering water and stir until melted.
3 Remove the bowl from the pan and beat the brandy into the chocolate mixture.
4 Stir in the dried fruits and nuts. Transfer the mixture to the pan and smooth to level the surface. Set aside to cool, then chill in the refrigerator until firm.
5 Cut into small bars or squares and serve on their own or with fresh fruit, such as strawberries and kiwi fruit for a delicious dessert.

variations

• *Use honey instead of maple syrup.*
• *Use whisky instead of brandy.*
• *Use chopped almonds and hazelnuts instead of Brazil nuts and cashews.*

fruit *with* strawberry sauce

This platter of fresh fruit served with a tangy strawberry sauce, is a rich source of vitamin C, which the body needs in greater amounts when under stress.

■ ingredients

- 8 ounces (225g) strawberries
- 1 tbsp honey
- 1–2 tsp cherry brandy or apple liqueur
- 1 small mango
- 2 apricots
- 1 kiwi fruit
- 2 papaya (or 1 medium-sized papaw)
- 4 fresh figs
- 4 ounces (115g) large, ripe blackberries
- fresh mint sprigs, to decorate

serves *four*
preparation time *20 minutes*

■ method

1 Put the strawberries in a blender or food processor and blend until smooth. Press the strawberry purée through a sieve and discard the seeds.
2 Pour the purée into a bowl. Add the honey and cherry brandy or liqueur and mix well. Cover and set aside.
3 Peel, pit, and slice the mango. Halve and pit the apricots, and peel and quarter the kiwi fruit. Peel, seed, and slice the papaya and quarter the figs.
4 Arrange the fresh fruit on a large serving platter. Decorate with fresh mint sprigs and serve with the strawberry coulis served separately in a jug alongside. Drizzle the coulis over individual servings of fruit.

variations

• *Use fresh ripe raspberries or blackberries instead of strawberries.*
• *Choose your own selection of fruit to serve on the platter.*

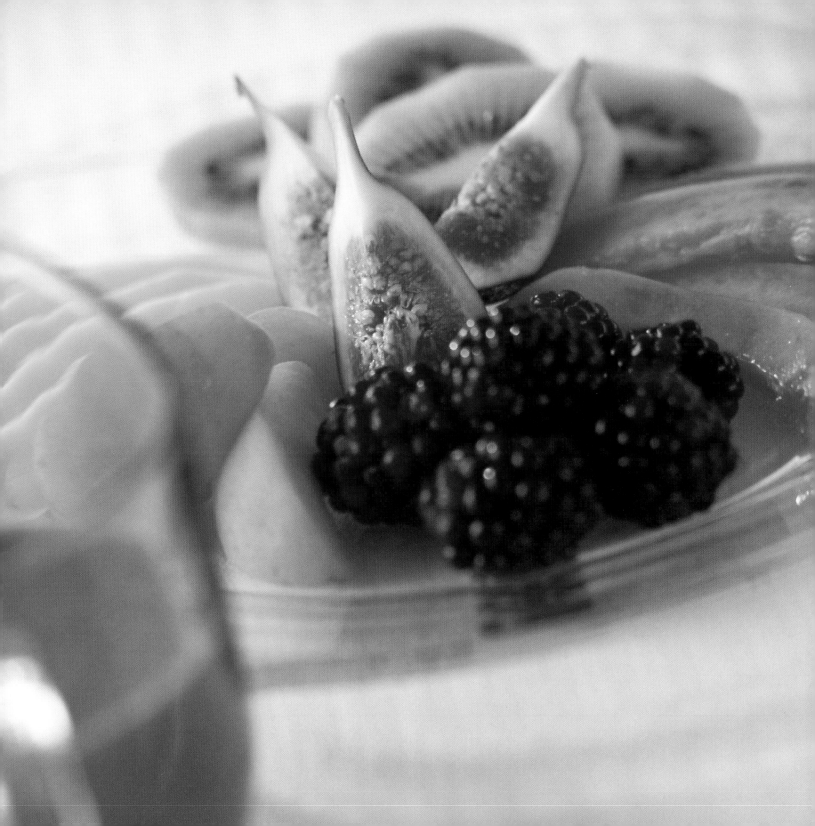

apricot upside-down pudding

This family favorite is delicious served with a little yogurt or homemade custard. Fresh, canned, and dried apricots contain many of the vitamins and minerals necessary for a healthy brain and nervous system.

ingredients

- 4tbsp maple syrup
- 1½ cups/6 ounces (175g) chopped, ready-to-eat dried apricots
- 1 8-ounce (220g) can apricots in fruit juice, drained and chopped
- ½ cup/4 ounces (115g) butter
- ½ cup/4 ounces (115g) light brown sugar
- 2 medium eggs, beaten
- 1½ cups/6 ounces (175g) whole-wheat flour
- 1 tsp baking powder
- 1 tsp ground cinnamon
- approx 3tbsp milk

serves *four to six*
preparation time *20 minutes*
cooking time *45 minutes*

method

1 Preheat the oven to 350°F.
2 Lightly grease and line a deep, 8-inch (20cm) round cake pan. Spoon or pour the maple syrup over the base.
3 Mix the dried and canned apricots, and scatter them evenly over the syrup. Set the pan aside.
4 Cream the butter and sugar in a bowl until pale and fluffy. Add the eggs gradually, beating after each addition.
5 Fold in the flour, baking powder, and cinnamon, adding enough milk to make a soft, dropping consistency. Spread the mixture evenly over the apricots and level the surface.
6 Bake for about 45 minutes, until the sponge has risen, and is springy to the touch, and golden brown.
7 Turn out onto a serving plate and serve hot or cold in wedges, with a little yogurt or homemade custard.

variations

- *Use dried and canned pears or peaches instead of apricots.*
- *Use honey instead of maple syrup.*
- *Use ground ginger or mixed spice instead of cinnamon.*

freezing instructions

Let cool completely; then wrap in foil, seal, and label. Freeze for up to 3 months. Defrost for several hours at room temperature. Reheat in a moderate oven.

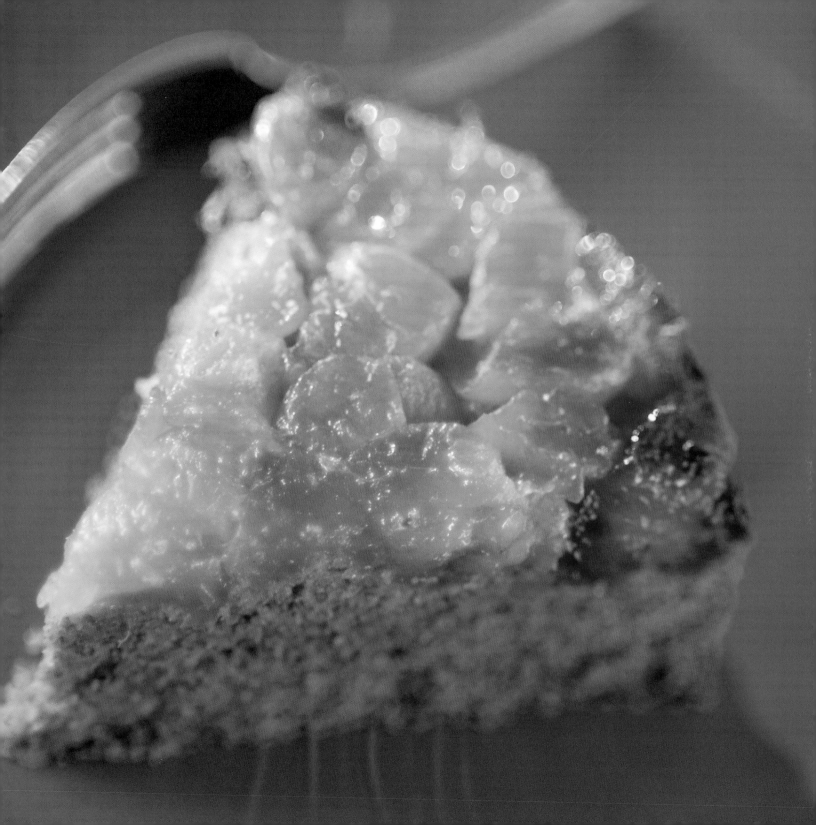

it's been a hard day's night

FLAGGING AFTER A HARD *day at the office? You need a quick fix of calming nutrients and comforting foods to help you unwind and* disperse *the feelings of tension—so tuck into this delicious menu from the reviving foods section for a dose of nutritional therapy.*

green bean vinaigrette

Green beans contain calcium, magnesium, and vitamin C.

ingredients

- 1½ pounds (700g) string beans, trimmed
- ⅔ cup/¼ pint (150ml) French dressing (see recipe on page 21)
- ½ cup/2 ounces (55g) toasted flaked almonds

serves *six*
preparation time *10 minutes*
cooking time *5–6 minutes*

method

1 Cook the beans in a large saucepan of lightly salted, boiling water for 5–6 minutes, until tender but still crisp. Drain well.
2 Serve the beans hot or cold, with the French dressing drizzled over the top. Sprinkle with flaked almonds just before serving.
3 Serve with crusty whole-wheat bread or bread rolls.

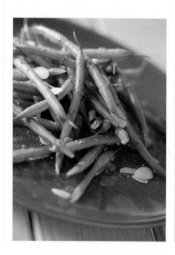

mediterranean vegetable lasagne

The complex carbo-hydrates in the pasta and vitamin C-rich vegetables are great stress relievers.

ingredients

- 1 onion, sliced
- 1 clove garlic, finely chopped
- 1 red bell pepper, seeded and sliced
- 1 yellow bell pepper, seeded and sliced
- 1 pound (450g) zucchini, sliced
- 12 ounces (350g) mushrooms, sliced
- 1 14-ounce (400g) can tomatoes, chopped
- 1 8-ounce (227g) can tomatoes, chopped
- 3 tbsp/1½ ounces (40g) butter
- 5 tbsp/1½ ounces (40g) whole-wheat flour
- ½ tsp mustard powder
- 2½ cups/1 pint (600ml) milk
- 1 cup/4 ounces (115g) Cheddar cheese, grated
- sea salt
- freshly ground black pepper
- 1–2 tbsp chopped, fresh mixed herbs
- 6 ounces (175g) lasagne noodles, cooked
- ¼ cup/1 ounce (25g) finely grated fresh Parmesan cheese
- fresh herb sprigs, to garnish

serves *four to six*
preparation time *25 minutes*
cooking time *45 minutes*

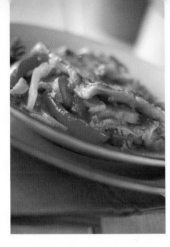

method

1 Preheat the oven to 350°F.

2 Put the onion, garlic, peppers, zucchini, mushrooms, and tomatoes in a large saucepan. Cover and simmer for 10 minutes, stirring occasionally.

3 Meanwhile, make the cheese sauce. Put the butter, flour, mustard powder, and milk in a saucepan and heat gently, whisking continuously, until the sauce comes to a boil and thickens. Simmer gently for 3 minutes.

4 Remove the pan from the heat and stir in the Cheddar cheese and seasoning, then the herbs.

5 Spoon half the vegetable mixture over the bottom of a shallow baking pan or ovenproof dish. Cover with half the pasta and top with one-third of the cheese sauce.

6 Repeat these layers, finishing with the remaining cheese sauce. Sprinkle with Parmesan cheese.

8 Bake for about 45 minutes, until cooked and golden brown on top.

9 Garnish with the herb sprigs and serve with whole-wheat bread and a mixed dark-green leaf salad.

apricot upside-down pudding

This warm, fruity, cake-like pudding is a comforting way to round off this soothing menu.

ingredients

- 4tbsp maple syrup
- 1½ cups/6 ounces (175g) chopped ready-to-eat dried apricots
- 1 8-ounce (220g) can apricots in fruit juice, drained and chopped
- ½ cup/4 ounces (115g) butter
- ½ cup/4 ounces (115g) light brown sugar
- 2 medium eggs, beaten
- 1½ cups/6 ounces (175g) whole-wheat flour
- 1tsp baking powder
- 1tsp ground cinnamon
- approx 3tbsp milk

serves *four to six*
preparation time *20 minutes*
cooking time *45 minutes*

method

1 Preheat the oven to 350°F.

2 Lightly grease and line a deep, 8-inch (20cm) round cake pan. Spoon or pour the maple syrup over the base.

3 Mix the dried and canned apricots, and scatter them evenly over the syrup. Set the pan aside.

4 Cream the butter and sugar in a bowl until pale and fluffy. Add the eggs gradually, beating after each addition.

5 Fold in the flour, baking powder, and cinnamon, adding enough milk to make a soft, dropping consistency. Spread the mixture evenly over the apricots and level the surface.

6 Bake for about 45 minutes, until the sponge has risen, and is springy to the touch, and golden brown.

7 Turn out onto a serving plate and serve hot or cold in wedges, with a little yogurt or homemade custard.

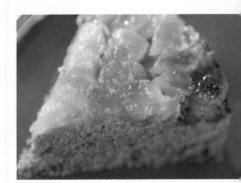

which mind problem *needs which* food?

poor sleep and insomnia

• Poor sleep can result from eating meals that are high in protein late at night. Protein foods such as eggs, cheese, meat, and poultry stimulate the mind and keep you awake. Complex carbohydrates such as cereals, rice, and pasta may help calm an over-active mind. A small bowl of muesli or oat-based cereal about an hour before bedtime can encourage sounder sleep.

• Insomnia is often a symptom of depression or stress, so while proper nutrition can help, it is also important to identify the root cause of any anxiety.

premenstrual syndrome

• Premenstrual syndrome may be related to a woman's changing hormone levels. To help with irritability, depression, and lethargy, some nutritionists recommend increasing the intake of foods that contain useful amounts of B6, such as meat, poultry, fish, wheat germ, cantaloupe, and green leafy vegetables. Research has shown that women who avoid sugar and caffeine and take regular exercise may experience a significant reduction in PMS.

problem

which mood problem *needs which* food?

stress

● When you are under stress, your body uses more vitamin C, which is vital for the production of the hormone noradrenalin, from the adrenal glands. Increase your intake of vitamin C by eating plenty of fresh fruit and vegetables, at least five portions a day. Top sources include oranges, grapefruit, kiwi fruit, lemons, bell peppers, tomatoes, and green leafy vegetables.

mood swings

● Mood swings, nervousness, anxiety, irritability, and apathy can result from a deficiency of B vitamins, which are essential to proper brain function. As all B vitamins work closely with each other, it is important to include them together in the diet. To get the widest range of B vitamins, include as many as possible of the following: apricots, avocado, bananas, melon, dried fruits, nuts, seeds, dark-green leafy vegetables, root vegetables, legumes, brown rice, oats, eggs and poultry, lean meats, seafood, and yogurt and other dairy products.

problem

vitamins *and* minerals

FOODS CONTAIN DIFFERENT *amounts of nutrients, and no single food can provide all the nutrients needed for good health. Vitamins and minerals found in foods work synergistically with proteins,* carbohydrates, fats, and each other. To make sure you obtain sufficient nutrients, vary your diet as much as possible. The following lists are a guide to recommended daily nutritional requirements.

Fat-soluble vitamins

vitamin A
from retinols in animal products or beta carotene in plant foods
Essential for growth and cell development, vision and immune function. Maintains healthy skin, hair, nails, bones, and teeth. Vital for immune function.

vitamin D
calciterol
Necessary for calcium absorption; helps to build and maintain strong bones and teeth.

vitamin E
tocopherols
Protects fatty acids; maintains muscles and red blood cells; a major antioxidant.

vitamin K
phylloquinone, menaquinone
Essential for proper blood clotting.

Water-soluble vitamins

biotin
Needed to release energy from food. Important in the synthesis of cholesterol, fat, and red blood cells.

folate
folic acid, folacin
Needed to make DNA, RNA, and red blood cells, and to synthesize certain amino acids.

niacin
vitamin B$_3$, nicotine acid, nictotinamide
Needed to metabolize energy; promotes normal growth.

pantothenic acid
vitamin B$_5$
Helps to release energy from food. Essential to the synthesis of cholesterol, fat, and red blood cells.

riboflavin
vitamin B$_2$
Needed to release energy from food and to assist the efficiency of vitamin B$_6$ and niacin.

thiamine
vitamin B$_1$
Needed to obtain energy from carbohydrates, fats, and alcohol; supports nerve function.

vitamin B$_6$
pyridoxine, pyridoxamine, pyridoxal
Help to release energy from proteins; important for immune function, the nervous system, and the formation of red blood cells.

vitamin B$_{12}$
cobalamins
Needed to make red blood cells, DNA, RNA, and myelin (for nerve fibers)

vitamin C
ascorbic acid
Vitamin C is a major antioxidant, vital for healthy immune function, which aids in the production of collagen, connective tissue, cartilage, and tendons. It is vital for wound healing, healthy gums, and the prevention of bruising.

Minerals

calcium
Builds strong bones and teeth; vital to muscle and nerve function, blood clotting, and metabolism.

magnesium
Stimulates bone growth; necessary for muscle function, metabolism, and nervous system.

phosphorus
Helps maintain strong bones and teeth. However, when taken to excess, it depletes calcium from the body.

chromium
Important for regulation of blood sugar levels; helps to regulate blood cholesterol levels and reduces cravings for junk foods.

copper
Needed for bone growth and connective tissue formation. Helps the body to absorb iron from food. Present in many enzymes that protect against free radicals.

iodine
Necessary to make thyroid hormones.

iron
Needed for the manufacture of red blood cells and for energy production within the cells.

manganese
Vital component of various enzymes involved in energy production; helps to form bone and connective tissue.

molybdenum
Essential component of enzymes involved in the production of DNA and RNA; may fight tooth decay.

selenium
A major antioxidant that works with vitamin E to protect cell membranes from oxidative damage. Very important for a healthy heart.

sulphur
Component of two essential amino acids that help to form many proteins in the body.

zinc
Essential for normal growth, reproduction, and immune function.

chloride
Maintains proper body chemistry. Used to make digestive juices.

potassium
Helps to maintain water balance and distribution, muscle and nerve function.

sodium
Works with potassium to regulate the body's fluid balance; promotes proper muscle function.

vitamins

US/CANADA

Recommended Dietary Allowances/Recommended Nutrient Intakes

(for adults over 24)

	MALES	FEMALES
Vitamin A	1000mcgR.E./1000mcgR.E.	800mcgR.E./800mcgR.E.
Vitamin D	5mcg/2.5mcg	5mcg/2.5mcg
Vitamin E	10mg/9mg	8mg/6mg
Vitamin K	80mcg/80mcg	65mcg/65mcg
Biotin	30–100mcg*/30–100mcg†	30–100mcg*/30–100mcg†
Folic acid	200mcg/230mcg	180mcg/185mcg
Vitamin B3	19mg/19mg	15mg/14mg
Vitamin B5	4–7mg*/4–7mg†	4–7mg*/4–7mg†
Vitamin B2	1.7mg/1.4mg	1.3mg/1mg
Vitamin B1	1.5mg/1.1mg	1.1mg/0.8mg
Vitamin B6	2mg/2mg†	1.6mg/1.6mg†
Vitamin B12	2mcg/1mcg	2mcg/1mcg
Vitamin C	60mg/40mg	60mg/40mg

* RDAs have not been established: values for these minerals are based on current expert opinion.
† RNIs have not been established: values for these minerals are based on current expert opinion.

minerals

US/CANADA

Recommended Dietary Allowances/Recommended Nutrient Intakes

(for adults over 24)

	MALES	FEMALES
Calcium	800mg/800mg	800mg/800mcg (1000–1500mg after menopause)
Magnesium	350mg/250mg	280mg/200mg
Phosphorus	800mg/1000mg	800mg/850mg
Chromium	0.05–0.2mg*/0.05–0.2mg†	0.05–0.2mg*/0.05–0.2mg†
Copper	1.5–3mg*/2–3mg†	1.5–3mg*/2–3mg†
Iodine	150mcg/160mcg	150mcg/160mcg
Iron	10mg/9mg	15mg/9–13mg
Manganese	2.5–5mg*/2.5–5mg†	2.5–5mg*/2.5–5mg†
Selenium	70mcg/70mcg	55mcg/55mcg
Zinc	15mg/12mg	12mg/9mg
Potassium	1875–5625mg*/2–6g†	1875–5625mg*/2–6g†
Sodium	1100–3300mg*/1–3g†	1100–3300mg*/1–3g†

* RDAs have not been established: values for these minerals are based on current expert opinion.
† RNIs have not been established: values for these minerals are based on current expert opinion.

index

A

alcohol, *8, 10*
alertness, *22, 44, 64, 84*
alfalfa sprouts, *15, 126*
almonds, *17, 58, 146, 166*
apples, *14, 40, 78, 80, 100, 120*
apricots, *14, 58, 100, 180, 182*
artichokes, globe, *15*
asparagus, *15, 26*
avocado, *10, 15, 44, 106*

B

bamboo shoots, *15*
bananas, *14, 58, 140*
barley, *16*
bean curd *see soybean curd*
beans, *8*
   broad, *138, 156*
   dried, *10, 16, 24, 56, 74, 113*
   green, *10, 15, 166*
bean sprouts, *15*
beets, *15*
bell peppers, *15, 110, 152, 158, 172, 174*
berry fruits, *14, 98, 162*
blackberries, *14, 40, 98, 162, 180*
blackcurrants, *14*
blackstrap molasses, *17*
blood sugar, *8–9, 13, 24, 104*
blueberries, *14, 98, 100, 162*
brain foods, *24–43*
brain function, *8, 9, 11, 13, 44, 64*
Brazil nuts, *17, 180*
breathing, *11*
broccoli, *10, 15, 28, 158*
buckwheat flour, *16*
butter, *11, 16*
buttermilk, *17*

C

cabbage, *15, 94, 136*
caffeine, *8, 10, 13*
calming foods, *10, 104–105, 106–125*
carambolas, *14, 80*
carbohydrates, *9, 10, 12, 106*
carrots, *15, 61, 86, 116, 136, 156*
cashew nuts, *17, 180*
cauliflower, *15, 94*
celery, *15, 30, 92, 136, 168*
cheese, *17, 126*
cherries, *14, 160, 162*

chicken
   main courses, *32, 52, 71, 92, 114, 154*
   nutritional value, *16*
   starters, *84, 128*
   stock, *20*
chocolate, *8, 78, 142, 180*
concentration, *22, 44, 64*
cooking times, *19*
corn, *10, 26*
couscous, *134*
cravings, *10*

D

dairy products, *16–17, 18*
dandelion leaves, *15*
desserts and bakes
   apple and apricot biscuit round, *100*
   apricot upside-down pudding, *182*
   banana and pecan muffins, *38*
   blackberry and apple streusel, *40*
   blueberry brûlée, *100*
   carrot and walnut cake, *61*
   cherry batter dessert, *160*
   chocolate, apple, and raisin cake, *78*
   date and raisin snack bars, *122*
   fresh figs with vanilla yogurt, *160*
   fruit, broiled with yogurt, *60*
   fruit, salad of golden, *38*
   fruit compote, *80*
   fruit and nut chocolate slices, *180*
   fruit salad with ginger, *122*
   fruit with strawberry sauce, *180*
   fruity florentines, *142*
   hazelnut meringues, *140*
   iced terrine of summer fruits, *162*
   peach and banana cream, *140*
   pineapple tarte tatin, *58*
   raspberry and apple oatmeal crumble, *120*
   triple berry cobbler, *98*
diet, *8–17*
digestion, *13*
duck, *174*

E

eggs, *10, 17, 18, 22, 47, 109, 128*
essential fatty acids, *9, 10–11, 12, 14, 18, 22–23*
exercise, *11*

F

fats, *8, 9, 10*
fiber, *10*
figs, *14, 160, 180*
fish, *10, 12, 16, 22*
   baked with lime and cilantro, *48*
   with broccoli sauce, *28*
   lemon sole, *88, 132*
   mackerel, *50, 152*
   oils, *10, 17*
   pilchards in herbed oatmeal, *112*
   salmon, *30, 110*
   trout, baked stuffed, *70*
   tuna, *130, 170*
fish *see also seafood*
French dressing, *21*
fruit, *10, 11, 14–15, 18, 23*
   dried, *14, 78, 94, 100, 122, 142, 180*
   fresh, *38, 60, 80, 122, 180*

G

garbanzo beans, *16, 52, 66, 178*
garlic, *15*
ginger, *15, 174*
grains, *1, 10, 12, 16, 18*
grapefruit, *14, 148*
grapes, *14*
guavas, *14*

H

hazelnuts, *17, 26, 140, 146*
herbs, *19*
honey, *17, 18, 32, 156*

I

ingredients, *9, 10, 18*

K

kelp, *15*
kidney beans, *10, 16, 56, 74, 113*
kiwi fruit, *14, 80, 122, 180*
kumquats, *14*

L

lamb, *16, 34, 51, 91, 134, 153*
lecithin, *23*
leek, *64, 95, 136, 173*
legumes, *10, 16*

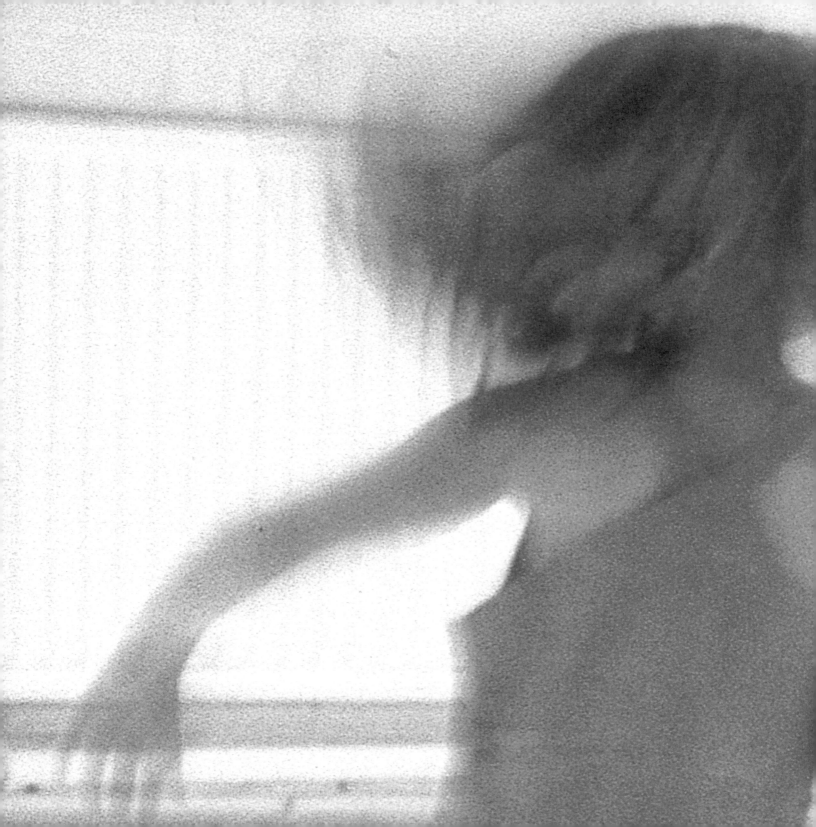